Michael D. Cardwell M.D.

Proceedings of a Brook Lodge Workshop

UTERINE PHYSIOLOGY

Proceedings of a Brook Lodge Workshop

UTERINE PHYSIOLOGY

Edited by
Emanuel A. Friedman, MD, ScD
Melvin L. Noah, MD
and
Bruce A. Work, Jr., MD

PSG Publishing Company, Inc.
Littleton, Massachusetts

Library of Congress Cataloging in Publication Data
Main entry under title:

Uterine physiology.

Workshop held at Brook Lodge, Augusta, Mich., on June 14, 1978.
1. Uterus, Pregnant—Congresses. 2. Labor (Obstetrics)—Congresses. I. Friedman, Emanuel A. II. Noah, Melvin L. III. Work, Bruce A.
[DNLM: 1. Labor—Congresses. 2. Uterus—Physiology—Congresses. 3. Uterine contraction—Congresses. WQ305 U89 1978]
RG655.U87 612.6'3 79-332
ISBN 0-88416-263-X

Printed in the United States of America.

International Standard Book Number: 0-88416-263-X

Library of Congress Catalog Card Number: 79-332

Acknowledgement

Continued support of medical research by
The Upjohn Company, Kalamazoo, Michigan,
has made this workshop possible.

Brook Lodge Workshop Participants

Mary E. Carsten, PhD
Professor
Department of Obstetrics and Gynecology
University of California, School of Medicine
Los Angeles

William H. Clewell, MD
Assistant Professor
Department of Obstetrics and Gynecology
University of Colorado Medical Center
Denver

Emanuel A. Friedman, MD, ScD
Professor
Department of Obstetrics and Gynecology
Harvard Medical School
Obstetrician-Gynecologist-in-Chief
Beth Israel Hospital
Boston, Massachusetts

Robert H. Hayashi, MD
Assistant Professor
Department of Obstetrics and Gynecology
University of Texas Health Science Center
San Antonio

Timothy J. Kriewall, PhD
Assistant Professor
Biomedical Engineering
The University of Michigan Medical School
Ann Arbor

Brook Lodge Workshop Participants

Melvin L. Noah, MD
Research Physician
Experimental Medical Research
The Upjohn Company
Kalamazoo, Michigan

Joseph Seitchik, MD
Professor and Chairman
Department of Obstetrics and Gynecology
The University of Texas Health Science Center
San Antonio

Stanley J. Stys, MD
Assistant Professor
Department of Obstetrics and Gynecology
The University of Cincinnati Medical Center
Cincinnati, Ohio

Bruce A. Work, Jr., MD
Associate Professor
Department of Obstetrics and Gynecology
The University of Michigan Medical School
Ann Arbor

CONTENTS

PREFACE

A vast amount of basic information has been generated concerning the function of the human gravid uterus and its mechanisms of action. Incomplete utilization of this store of knowledge has resulted in little of it finding application to clinical problems. An intensive workshop was conducted at Brook Lodge, Augusta, Michigan, on June 14, 1978, aimed at making an attempt to bridge the wide gap between basic laboratory science and clinical practice. Our collective objective was to provide insights into relevant matters of critical interest in our discipline, specifically as they relate to labor phenomena.

Because so many important areas were identified, it was agreed that the proceedings of the workshop would undoubtedly prove beneficial to both scientist and clinician working in this field. This volume is dedicated to the goal of disseminating these perspectives. The participants and discussants have made a concerted effort to examine our shared problems, first in overview and then in close focus. In this way, they portray the broad sweep of unresolved issues while at the same time offering areas of potential solution for possible fruitful research in the laboratory or the clinical setting.

We are encouraged by the emphasis that has been made to delineate the frontiers of and new developments in physiologic and physiopathologic mechanisms, seeking to provide better understanding of the labor process by researchers as well as clinicians, each perhaps from the other's vantage. We thus share factual material and newer concepts that have evolved as a consequence of the research activities which we reviewed together. Much deals with work still in progress, lending an air of immediacy to the discussions. In order to derive optimal return, we enjoin the reader to steep himself or herself in the spirit of our profitable interchange.

We are grateful to all the participants who gave of themselves so unstintingly and with such enthusiasm and energy. Without their strong motivation the workshop would not have been nearly so successful in achieving its aims. We are also grateful to The Upjohn Company for having provided the wherewithal to make the meeting possible. Support was given without exerting either overt or subtle pressures on its organizers to modify the program or the contributors so as to yield any direct benefit whatsoever. We are most appreciative.

Emanuel A. Friedman

1 Introduction

Bruce A. Work, Jr.

The format we have chosen here is meant to provide a framework for discussion among individuals with diversified expertise. Clinicians and researchers from widely varying disciplines have been brought together in an isolated yet comfortable setting in an effort to catalyze interchange. We desire to cross-fertilize our several disciplines so as to provide insight that may in due course lead to solutions to unresolved dilemmas that some of us face daily in our clinical practices.

We are hopeful that the formal presentations will serve merely as the starting points and foci for stimulating and informative discussions. We seek genuine dialogues among participants. Our aim would ideally be to keep the proceedings unstructured, but of course some structure is necessary. We wish to deal with facts and ideas, and particularly to generate thoughts about those avenues of investigation that might be embarked upon with reasonable prospects of success in helping to unravel knotty problems for us. The sequence of subjects should not be rigidly constraining insofar as discussions are concerned, although we have designed a more or less logical development.

To begin with, some critical aspects of basic uterine physiology will be reviewed, concentrating on two broad areas of special interest in parturition, namely, the biochemistry of contractility and the mechanisms for control of uterine circulation. Then we will pursue recent developments in research dealing with the changes that the cervix undergoes in labor.

Following this, we will delve into some areas of applied physiology. Attention will be directed at means for assessing the waveforms of intrauterine pressure as a diagnostic tool. We will conclude the formal presentations with a most important offering on the effects that may result from the forces of labor when they act upon the cervix and upon the fetal skull.

2 Biochemical Aspects of Uterine Contractility: Role of Prostaglandins

Mary E. Carsten

The last few years have seen the development of prostaglandins (PG) as a tool in clinical obstetrics. Its mode of action is still largely unknown, but its first and primary effect appears to be on uterine contraction. In my laboratory, we have studied some interactions of PG with its target organ, the myometrium. I will share with you today our progress in this area and some of our problems and thoughts. In order to place this work in the proper perspective, we will deal with the subject in three segments. The first is on uterine muscle. The second will be a discussion of our findings on the interactions of PG, oxytocin, and progesterone with cellular constituents of the myometrium. Prostaglandins will be discussed because of their role in the onset of parturition and the maintenance of labor, as well as their clinical usefulness in pregnancy termination. Oxytocin will be studied because of its involvement in the onset of labor and its use in labor induction. Progesterone is an important component because of its blocking action on the

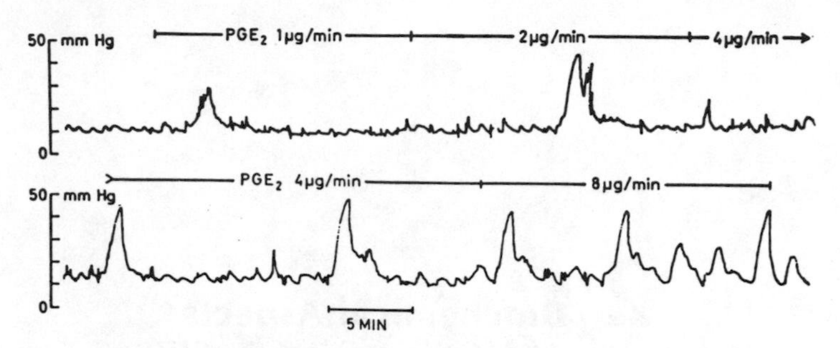

Figure 1. The uterine dose-response to intravenous infusion of PGE_2 in a term pregnant patient. From Bygdeman, M., Kwon, S.U., Mukherjee, T., and Wiqvist, N. *Am. J. Obstet. Gynecol.* 102:317, 1968.

uterus. The third section will deal with some physiologic implications of our findings.

The effect of PG on the uterus in a term pregnant patient is shown in Figure 1. It goes without saying, as we all know, that the uterus contracts. We recognize that more frequent and stronger contractions occur with increasing doses of PG. Our initial hypothesis was that because PG is a contractile agent, it should act directly with the contractile machinery of the cell.

To help us understand this mechanism, let us first look at a diagram of a smooth muscle cell (Figure 2). This cell is different from nonmuscle cells inasmuch as it contains actin and myosin filaments. These proteins represent the contractile mechanism. In relaxation, the thin actin filament and the thick myosin filament are separate. In contraction, actin and myosin combine. Myosin is an adenosine triphosphatase (ATPase) which is strongly activated when myosin is combined with actin. ATPase is split to provide the energy for contraction. This reaction requires Mg^{++} and a trace of Ca^{++}.

The contractile mechanism is essentially very similar to that which pertains in skeletal muscle, although there are subtle differences with respect to the regulatory factors involved. The question of these regulatory factors as related to smooth muscle contraction is presently subject to a great deal of controversy. It is certain, however, that a regulatory protein and calcium are required for contraction.

The amounts of calcium required in these reactions are exceedingly small. The contractile elements are activated

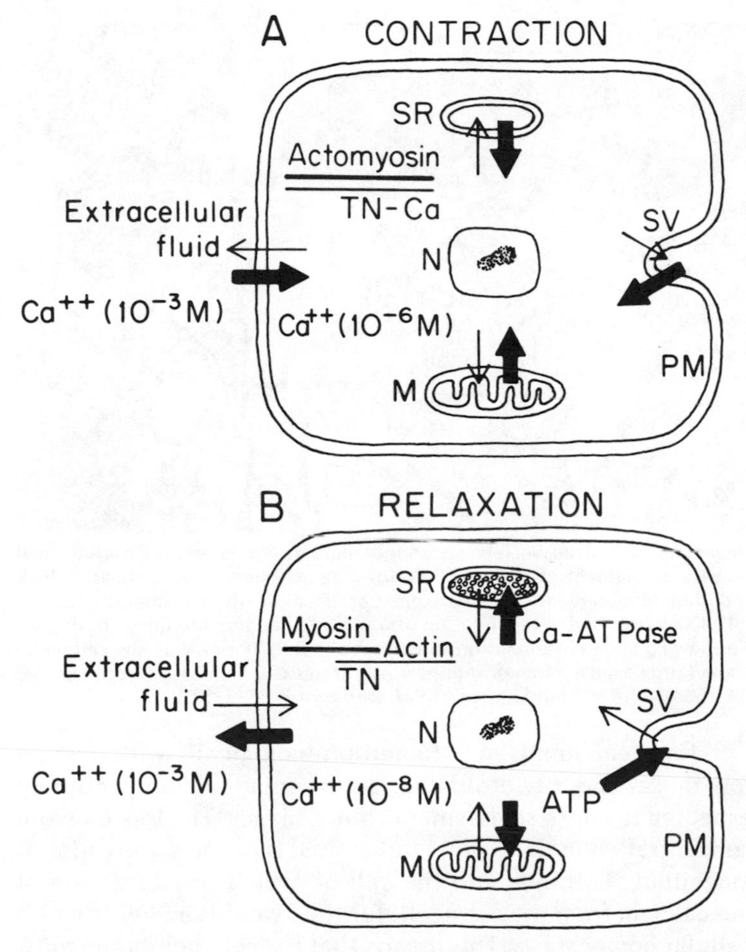

Figure 2. Cellular calcium movements determining uterine contraction and relaxation. Heavy arrows indicate predominant direction of calcium flow. A: Passive release of calcium to activate contraction from sarcoplasmic reticulum (SR), mitochondria (M), plasma membrane (PM), and surface vesicles (SV), in association with movement of extracellular fluid into the interior of the cell. B: Energy-requiring processes of calcium uptake into structural elements and efflux across the plasma membrane for relaxation. TN, troponin.

when intracellular free calcium rises above 10^{-7} M, and activation is maximal at 10^{-6} M. In relaxation, the intracellular calcium concentration falls to 10^{-8} M. Serum calcium concentration is 4.77 mEq/l; half of this calcium is ionized (10^{-3} M).

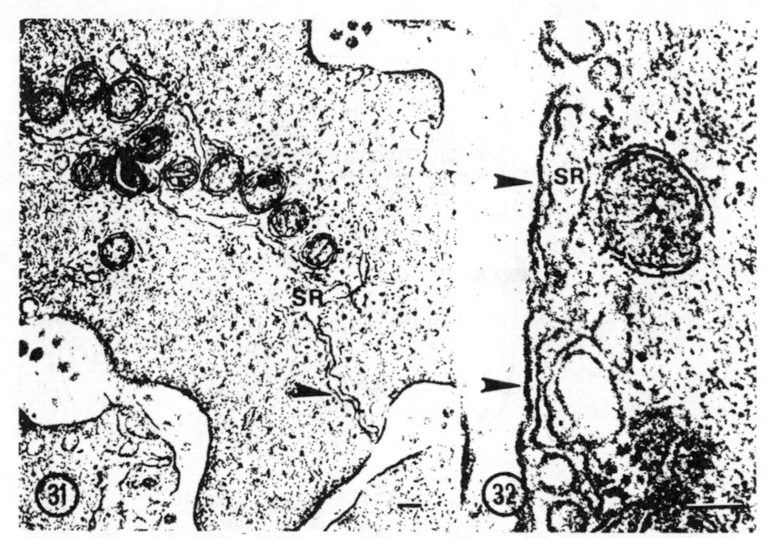

Figure 3. Left: Transversely sectioned human uterine smooth muscle cell showing an element of central SR continuing peripherally (arrowhead). Thick and thin myofilaments are also present. Human uterine smooth muscle, × 42,400. Right: High magnification of a region of human uterine smooth muscle showing SR in close relationship (approximately 10 nm) with the cell membrane (arrowheads). Human uterine smooth muscle, × 103,500. From Devine, C.E., Somlyo, A.V., and Somlyo, A.P. *J. Cell Biol.* 52:690, 1972.

Ionic calcium is maintained physiologically within a narrow range, and a twofold change in serum calcium would be expected to cause severe metabolic changes. The free calcium concentration in the extracellular fluid is of the same order of magnitude. Entrance into the cell of even a small fraction of the calcium from the extracellular fluid would severely disturb cellular homeostasis. This means that the cell membrane must support an approximately 10,000-fold concentration gradient.

Activator calcium is supplied from both outside and inside the cell. This is supported by the following evidence. First, in smooth muscle the calcium current is very low. The amount of calcium that enters the cell with an action potential is insufficient to activate the contractile state fully.[1] Second, with calcium efflux blocked, some contracted smooth muscles are still able to relax.[2] Both these observations imply the existence of intracellular calcium binding and/or storage sites.

In smooth muscle, the intracellular structures potentially capable of supplying activator calcium are plasma membrane

$$E + n\mathrm{Ca}^{2+} \rightleftharpoons E(\mathrm{Ca})_n$$

$$E(\mathrm{Ca})_n + \mathrm{ATP} \rightleftharpoons \mathrm{P}E(\mathrm{Ca})_n + \mathrm{ADP}$$

$$\mathrm{P}E(\mathrm{Ca})_n \rightleftharpoons \mathrm{P}E^*(\mathrm{Ca})_n$$

$$\mathrm{P}E^*(\mathrm{Ca})_n + \mathrm{Mg}^{2+} \rightleftharpoons \mathrm{P}E^*(\mathrm{Mg}) + n\mathrm{Ca}^{2+}$$

$$\mathrm{P}E^*(\mathrm{Mg}) \rightleftharpoons E + \mathrm{P}_1 + \mathrm{Mg}^{2+}$$

Figure 4. ATPase reaction coupled with calcium transport. From Hidalgo, C., Ikemoto, N., and Gergely, J. *J. Biol. Chem.* 251:14, 1976.

(PM) and its surface vesicles (SV), sarcoplasmic reticulum (SR), mitochondria (M), and the cell nucleus. In contraction, calcium moves into the cell from outside and calcium is released from storage sites in the SR and possibly from sites in the M, the PM and its SV. In relaxation, the opposite takes place: calcium is taken up into the SR, possibly into the M, the PM and SV, and calcium is extruded into the extracellular fluid. The uptake and extrusion of calcium in relaxation requires energy in the form of ATP. Thus, ATP is needed in contraction for the actin-myosin interaction and in relaxation for calcium pump activity.

The relative importance of the various intracellular organelles is still unknown. But the role of the SR as a calcium-accumulating site is well documented by a variety of lines of evidence, such as electron microscopy,[3] histochemical studies,[4] x-ray spectra,[4] and electron probe analysis.[5] The amount of SR differs in different kinds of smooth muscle and correlates with the ability of the muscle to contract in the absence of extracellular calcium.[3] In the human uterus, SR is relatively abundant (Figure 3). In skeletal muscle, SR is established as the main intracellular calcium storage site. The chemical reaction sequence (Figure 4) in the SR is as follows. In relaxation, an ATPase enzyme located in the membranes of the SR binds calcium. The enzyme-calcium complex is phosphorylated while splitting ATP to ADP. A conformational change in the phosphorylated enzyme-calcium complex results in exchange of calcium for magnesium. Calcium is released inside the vesicles. Finally, dissociation into enzyme, Mg, and P occurs.

As to other organelles (Figure 2), mitochondria may be the main calcium storage site in smooth muscle cells. However, in view of their topography and their relatively low rate of calcium uptake at low calcium concentration,[6] they do not appear to be a source of *activator* calcium. The role of the nucleus in intracellular calcium homeostasis is unclear. Surface vesicles occupy large areas of the smooth muscle cell membrane and were shown to contain a Ca-ATPase.[4] This ATPase must function physiologically by pumping calcium out of the cell.

HORMONES AS REGULATING AGENTS

Since uterine contractility is regulated by intracellular calcium levels, we propose that the uterine contractile action of PG may consist in regulating cellular calcium movements. In my laboratory, we have attempted to demonstrate effects of PG on the calcium-accumulating system of the uterus. In this regard, we have focused on the SR.

Modifying methods employed for isolating SR from cardiac muscle, we have isolated a subcellular fraction from bovine and human uterus. Differential centrifugation (15,000 to 40,000 g) followed by sucrose density gradient centrifugation yields a microsomal fraction enriched in SR.[7] This microsomal fraction is of vesicular nature and takes up calcium from solution in the presence of ATP. The amount of calcium bound amounts to approximately 24 nmol Ca per mg protein per 8 minutes at 37°C in our present preparations.

The microsomal fraction appears free of mitochondria, an important consideration since calcium uptake is not inhibited by agents which inhibit mitochondrial calcium uptake, such as sodium azide and dicumarol. However, possible contamination with plasma membrane fragments cannot be excluded. We have also demonstrated a Ca, Mg-ATPase.[7] In our in vitro system, calcium accumulation in microsomes would be equivalent to in vivo relaxation, as free calcium is removed from solution; and calcium release, which increases the free calcium concentration, would make calcium available for contraction.

We investigated two contractile agents (PG and oxytocin) and one relaxing agent (progesterone) as to their effect on calcium accumulation. Microsomal preparations were incubated in a calcium-containing medium in the presence and absence of ATP for one minute. The difference in calcium associated with the microsomes is the ATP-dependent calcium binding.

We then designed experiments to see whether addition of PG would change the amount of calcium bound (Figure 5). Graded amounts of PGE_2, $PGF_{2\alpha}$ (contractile), and $PGF_{1\beta}$ (inactive) were added to the incubation mixtures. These initial experiments were done on preparations from nonpregnant bovine uterus.[8] Figure 5 shows percent inhibition of ATP-dependent calcium binding in the presence of the three PG preparations. We found that PGE_2 and $PGF_{2\alpha}$ inhibited ATP-dependent calcium binding in a log dose-response fashion. This inhibition was found to be statistically highly significant ($p<0.005$), using Student's t test in paired comparisons. $PGF_{1\beta}$, a

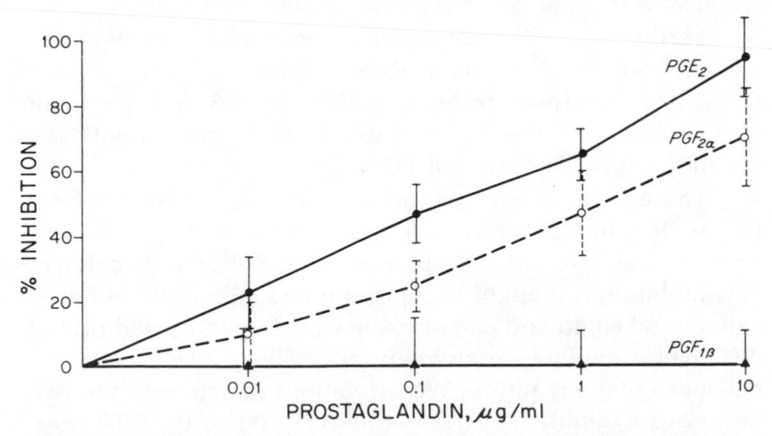

Figure 5. Inhibition of ATP-dependent calcium binding by PGE_2, $PGF_{2\alpha}$, and $PGF_{1\beta}$ in preparations from nonpregnant bovine uterus. Vertical bars represent ±SEM. From Carsten, M.E. In N.L. Stephens (Ed.). *The Biochemistry of Smooth Muscle.* Baltimore: University Park Press, 1977, p. 617.

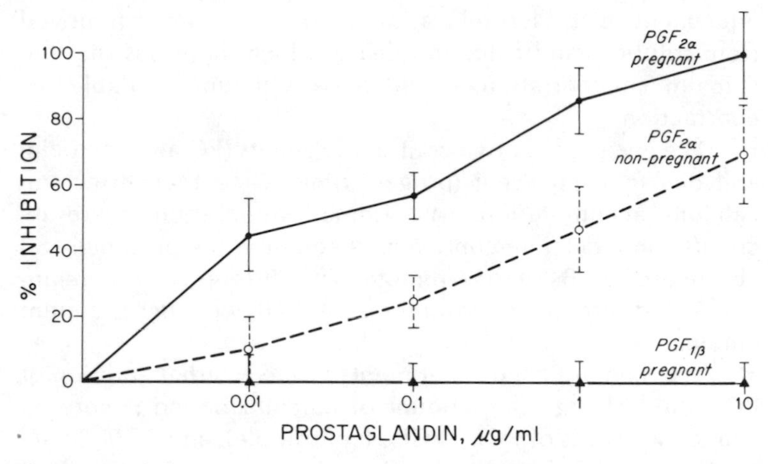

Figure 6. Inhibition of ATP-dependent calcium binding by $PGF_{2\alpha}$ in preparations from pregnant and nonpregnant bovine uterus; $PGF_{1\beta}$ in preparations from pregnant uterus. From Carsten, M.E. *Prostaglandins* 5:33, 1974.

physiologically inactive analogue, did not elicit any response. The inhibition with $PGF_{2\alpha}$ was less complete than with PGE_2. Statistical analysis by Student's t distribution showed a significant difference in the effect of PGE_2 and $PGF_{2\alpha}$. These results suggest that there is a difference in the magnitude of the effectiveness of PGE_2 and $PGF_{2\alpha}$ on the cellular level.

Furthermore, SR from the pregnant uterus (Figure 6) was more sensitive to $PGF_{2\alpha}$ than SR from the nonpregnant uterus.[8] $PGF_{1\beta}$ had no effect on SR preparations from the pregnant uterus either. All these observations are in accord with the uterine contractile action of PG.

These findings led to a further question. Does PG inhibit the binding of calcium to the SR vesicles or does it induce calcium release? In SR preparations, observed calcium accumulation is thought to represent an equilibrium between calcium taken up and calcium released. Repeated addition of ATP will stimulate calcium uptake. Thus, ATP favors the calcium uptake reaction. We attempted to separate the two processes by limiting the available ATP. When the ATP is exhausted, a steady state of calcium should prevail in the SR preparations. PG added at this point could then cause calcium release only.

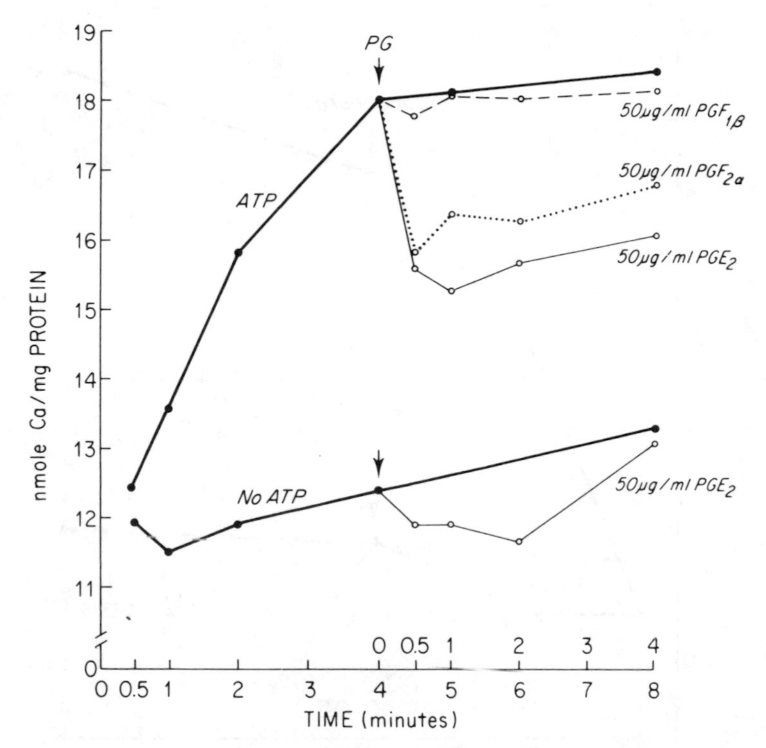

Figure 7. Calcium release. Incubation medium consists of 20 mM imidazole buffer, pH 7.0, 0.15 mM ATP, 0.15 mM $MgCl_2$, 10 mM KCL, 20 µM $CaCl_2$, and 0.5 mg/ml of microsomal protein. Prostaglandins E_2, $F_{2\alpha}$, $F_{1\beta}$ added at arrow. Prostaglandin concentration in the incubation medium, 50 µg/ml. From Carsten, M.E., and Miller, J.D. *J. Biol. Chem.* 252:5, 1977.

In these experiments (Figure 7), SR was preloaded with calcium.[7] The ATP concentration was limited to 0.15 mM. A steady state of calcium was obtained in the microsomes when the ATP was exhausted after four minutes. Addition of PGE_2 or $PGF_{2\alpha}$ at this point caused release of calcium. PGE_2 appeared to be more powerful than $PGF_{2\alpha}$, but this difference was statistically not significant. $PGF_{1\beta}$ was ineffective. The PG released only calcium previously taken up in the presence of ATP and had no effect on calcium initially present in the SR preparations. However, higher concentrations of PG were needed to enhance calcium release than to inhibit ATP-dependent calcium binding in previous experiments.

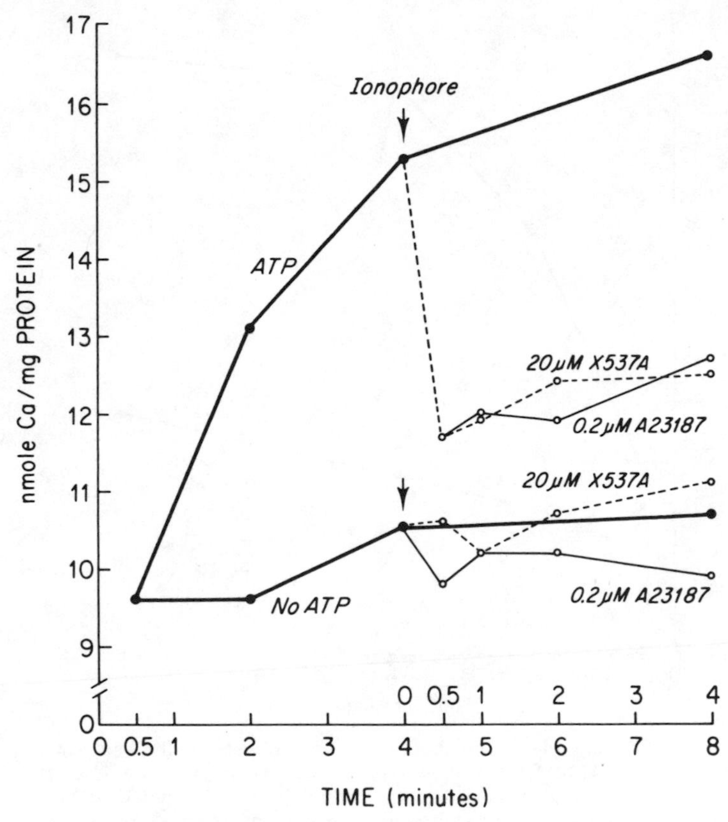

Figure 8. Effect of ionophores on calcium release. Incubation medium as in Figure 7. Ionophores X537A (20 μM) and A23187 (0.2 μM) were added at arrow. From Carsten, M.E., and Miller, J.D. *J. Biol. Chem.* 252:5, 1977.

How do these hormones work? One hypothesis we have advanced is that PG may act as an ionophore.[7] Ionophores are substances that modify membrane permeability to specific ions by forming ion complexes and carrying the ion complexes across a membrane to release the ion at the opposite interface. Some bacterial polypeptides are recognized ionophores and have been shown to potentiate the twitch force of single muscle fibers, to contract some smooth muscles, and to release calcium from SR preparations of skeletal muscle. We can show (Figure 8) that the ionophores A23187 (Eli Lilly) and X537A (Hoffmann-La Roche) cause release of calcium from preloaded microsomal preparations.

Prostaglandins are water and lipid soluble and form calcium complexes; they therefore appear to be well suited for calcium transport. If the PG-calcium complexes are highly soluble in lipid layers (Table 1), the PG may transport calcium across biological membranes, such as those of the SR vesicles. A prerequisite for transporting calcium is that the PG should form calcium complexes. Hence, we measured the PG-calcium association constants.[9] We found them much lower than those of the ionophores.

Table 1
Molar Association Constants of Calcium Complexes*

	PGB_2	PGE_2	A23187	X537A
$K_a \pm SEM (M^{-1})$	359 ± 12.4	326 ± 18.1	27,444 ± 3,907	2,695 ± 107
Number of data points	11	12	6	6

*From Carsten, M.E., and Miller, J.D. *Arch. Biochem. Biophys.* 185:282, 1978.

Next we used a modified Pressman cell as a bulk phase transport system (Figure 9). Siliconized flat bottom tubes were layered with 1.5 ml buffered 30% (w/v) sucrose containing 10 mM $CaCl_2$ with ^{45}Ca (bottom); 1.5 ml of organic phase containing a test compound (center); and 1.5 ml buffer with 10 mM

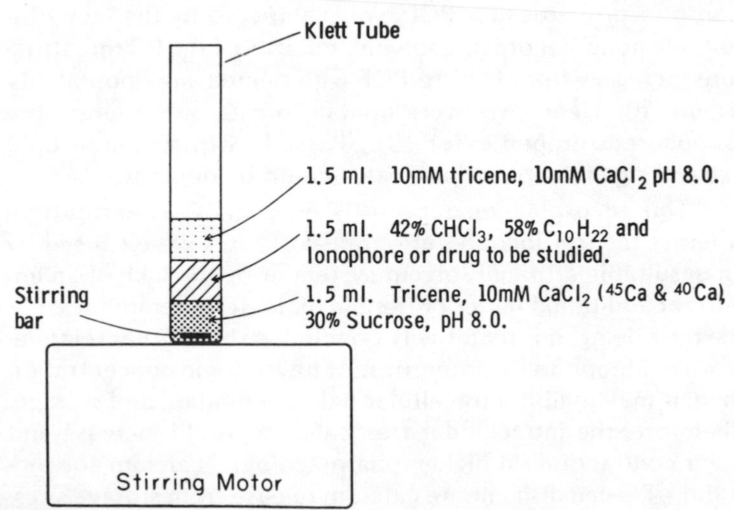

Figure 9. Vertically stacked bulk phase transport system.

$CaCl_2$ (top). Organic phase was chloroform:decane (42:52). The bottom solution was mechanically stirred. Samples were removed from the top for counting after constant transport rates had been established (Table 2). We demonstrated that the ionophores X537A and A23187 were capable of transporting calcium through organic solvent layers.

Table 2
Transport Rates for Calcium Complexes*

	Nanomoles of Ca^{2+} per hour				
	pH 8.0				
	Blank	X537A (1×10^{-4}M)	A23187 (1×10^{-4}M)	PGB_2 (1×10^{-3}M)	PGE_2 (1×10^{-3}M)
Mean	0.0264	27.5	32.3	1.66	0.067
±SEM	±0.009	±0.178	±0.856	±0.315	±0.037
Number of trials	23	36	31	32	33
P		0.0005	0.0005	0.0005	0.15

*From Carsten, M.E., and Miller, J.D. *Arch. Biochem. Biophys.* 185:282, 1978.

Similar calcium transport could be demonstrated for PGB_2; however, the transport rate for PGE_2, a PG with highly polar properties, was only marginal. The observation of transport properties for PGE_2 was hampered by the lack of a suitable nonpolar organic solvent. Polarity of the PG ring structure increases from PGB to PGF with decreasing lipophilicity (Figure 10). Hence, we were unable to establish appreciable ionophoretic properties for PGE_2. Possibly, with a suitable lipid extract, significant transport rates could be demonstrated.

Thus, in explaining our results, we cannot say at this time whether the low ionophoretic transport rates were caused by an unsuitable artificial solvent system or by the lack of an important additional factor present in biological membranes. For the time being, it is tentatively concluded that PG has relatively weak ionophoretic properties. At physiologic concentration then, it may inhibit intracellular calcium binding and storage. Therefore, the intracellular free calcium would increase and favor contraction. At higher (pharmacologic) calcium concentration, PG can also initiate calcium release from storage sites,

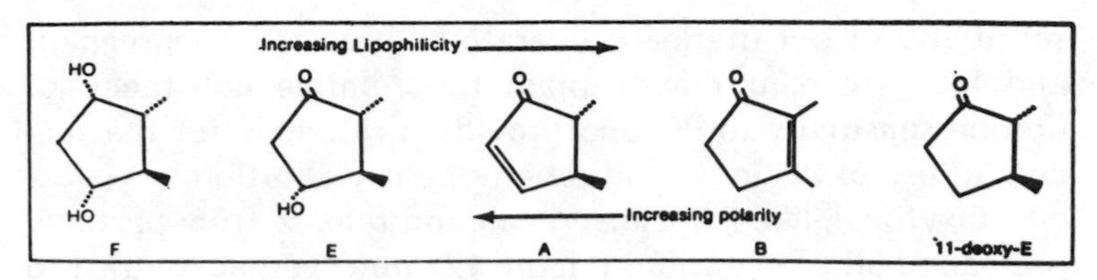

Figure 10. Polarity of different prostaglandin ring structures. From Andersen, N.H., and Ramwell, P.W. *Arch. Intern. Med.* 133:30, 1974.

possibly by acting as ionophores. Clearly, more work is needed on this problem.

The second contractile agent investigated was oxytocin. Oxytocin was added to incubation media in experiments analogous to those performed with PG (Figure 11). We found that oxytocin, like PG, inhibited ATP-dependent calcium binding in a dose dependent fashion.[8]

The pregnant bovine uterus at term was found to be very much more sensitive to oxytocin than the nonpregnant uterus. The increased sensitivity of the gravid term uterus was still more pronounced in response to oxytocin than to $PGF_{2\alpha}$. The mechanism for this could be either increased numbers of receptors in the pregnant uterus, or a direct effect of the hormones on the transport ATPase, or both. At any rate, the findings for oxytocin agree with the known increase in reactivity to oxytocin of the bovine and the human uterus in advanced pregnancy.

The situation for oxytocin thus is clearer than for PG, although during the menstrual cycle changes in human uterine sensitivity to PG have been reported. The *small* difference in

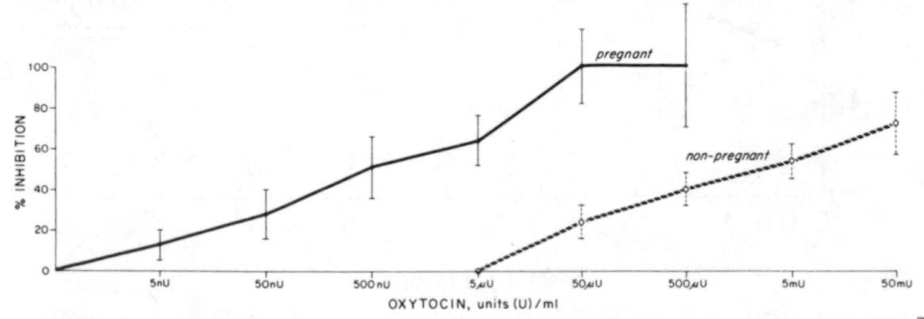

Figure 11. Inhibition of ATP-dependent calcium binding by oxytocin in preparations from pregnant and nonpregnant uterus. From Carsten, M.E. *Prostaglandins* 5:33, 1974.

sensitivity of our uterine preparations between nonpregnant and late pregnant may explain the relative constancy of uterine sensitivity to PG and provide a rationale for the successful use of PG in the induction of early abortion.

Oxytocin, like PG, caused calcium release from partially preloaded SR preparations (Figure 12); however, in contrast to PG, oxytocin also released intrinsic calcium.[7] It appears that

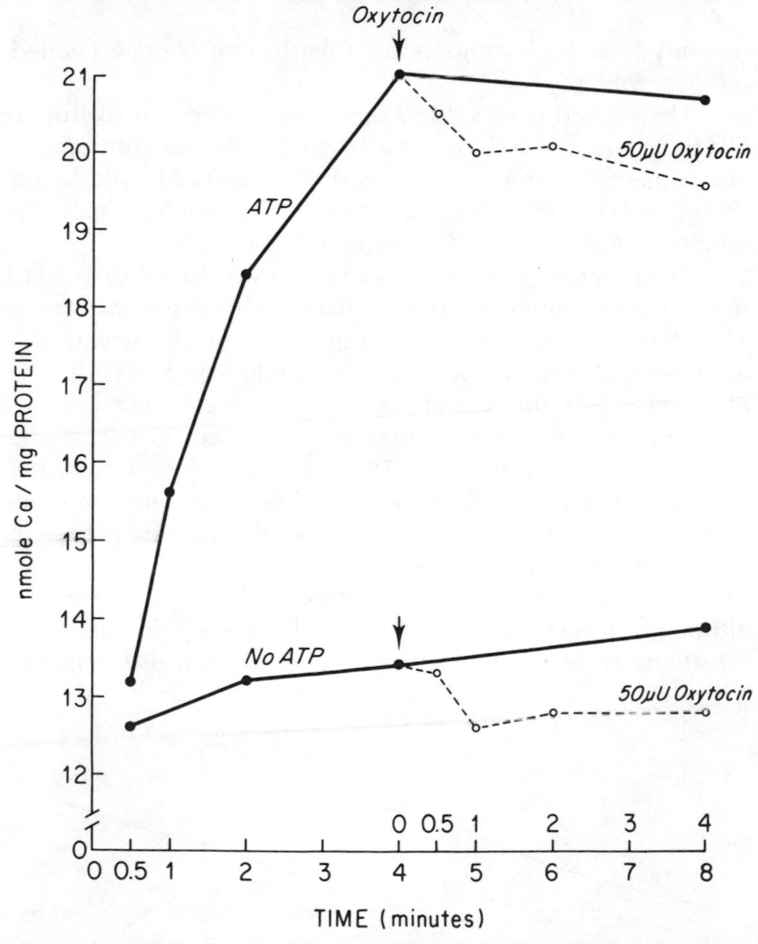

Figure 12. Effect of oxytocin on calcium release. Incubation medium as in Figure 7. Oxytocin added at arrow, 50 μU/ml of incubation medium. From Carsten, M.E., and Miller, J.D. *J. Biol. Chem.* 252:5, 1977.

the physiologic effect of oxytocin is consistent with its inhibition of calcium binding, but may not be due to release of calcium from calcium stores accumulated in the presence of ATP. Thus, the mode of action of oxytocin in releasing calcium appears to be different from that of PG and the ionophores.

In other experiments both $PGF_{2\alpha}$ and oxytocin were added to incubation mixtures in calcium uptake studies to see whether their effects were additive (Figure 13). We found that, in the presence of both $PGF_{2\alpha}$ and oxytocin, inhibition of calcium accumulation was further increased in comparison to the inhibition with either hormone alone. The data do not allow us to conclude whether $PGF_{2\alpha}$ enhances the effect of

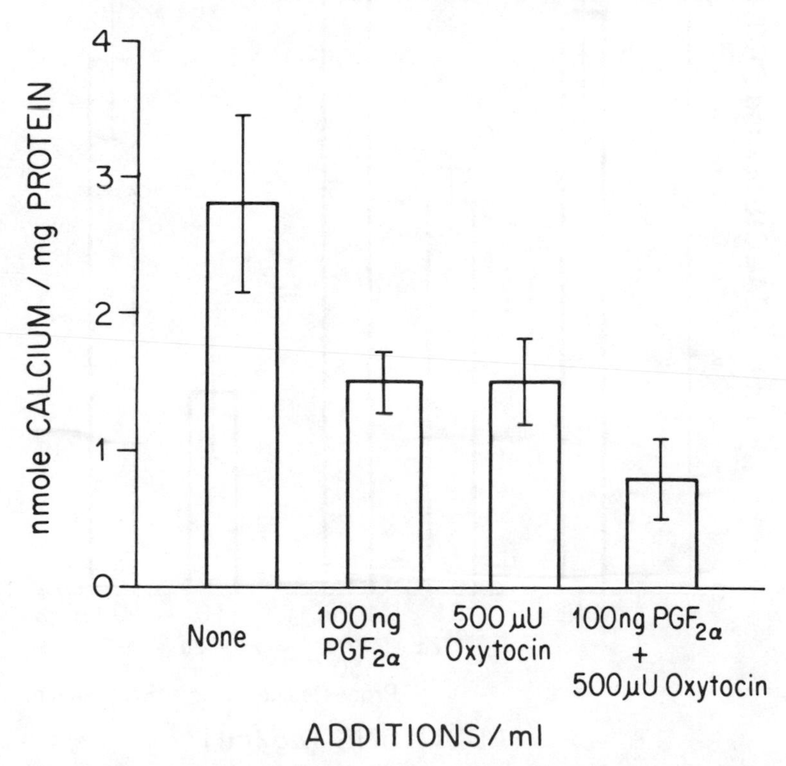

Figure 13. Inhibition by $PGF_{2\alpha}$ and oxytocin of ATP-dependent calcium binding in nonpregnant bovine uterus. From Carsten, M.E. In N.L. Stephens (Ed.). *The Biochemistry of Smooth Muscle.* Baltimore: University Park Press, 1977, p. 617.

oxytocin or vice versa. These experiments were carried out because of claims of beneficial effects of a combination of $PGF_{2\alpha}$ and oxytocin in the induction of labor.

Experiments with progesterone were designed to test the

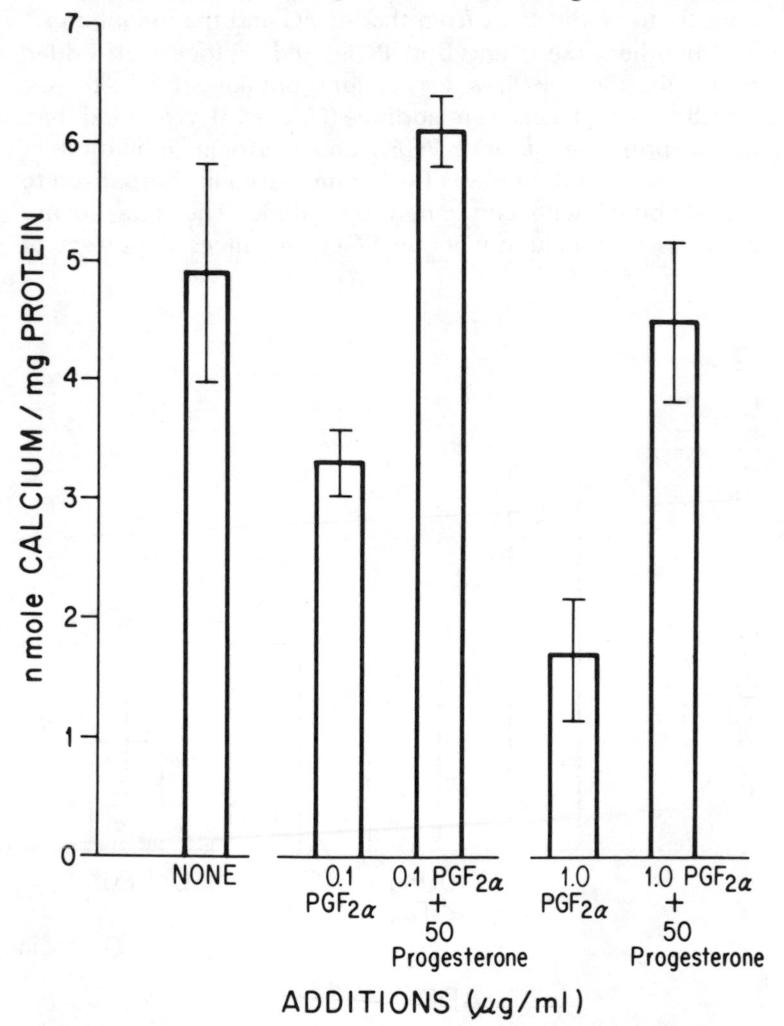

Figure 14. Effects of progesterone and $PGF_{2\alpha}$ on ATP-dependent calcium binding in nonpregnant bovine uterus. From Carsten, M.E. In N.L. Stephens (Ed.). *The Biochemistry of Smooth Muscle*. Baltimore: University Park Press, 1977, p. 617.

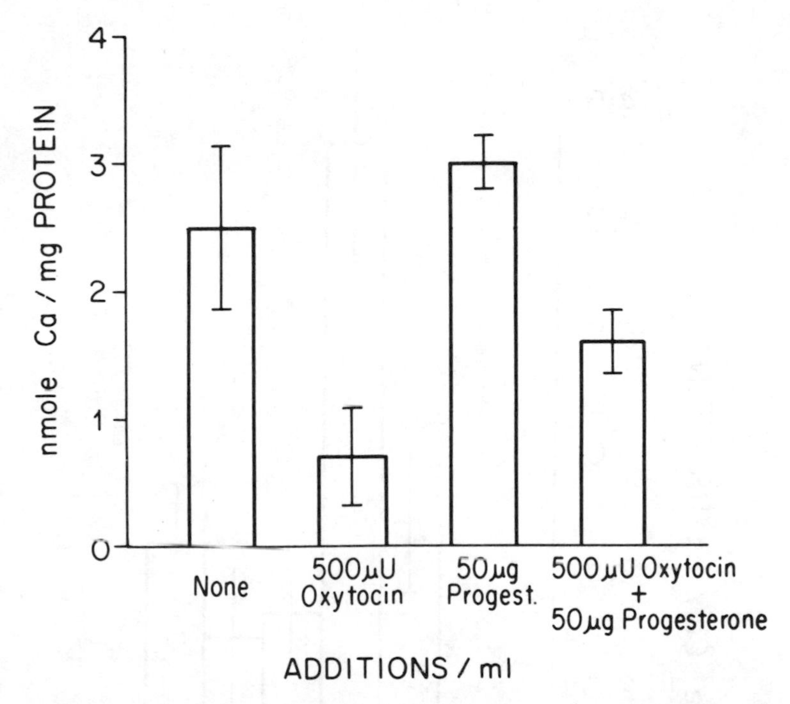

Figure 15. ATP-dependent calcium binding in the presence of oxytocin and progesterone. From Carsten, M.E. *Gynecol. Invest.* 5:269, 1974.

hypothesis that progesterone has a blocking action on the uterus by blocking calcium movement and limiting the availability of calcium for contraction.[10] If our hypothesis is correct, progesterone should increase ATP-dependent calcium binding and oppose the effects of PG and oxytocin.

Progesterone added to incubation media increased ATP-dependent calcium accumulation and antagonized the effects of prostaglandins on ATP-dependent calcium binding (Figure 14). Similarly, progesterone counteracted the oxytocin effect (Figure 15). The progesterone effect was specific. Three known metabolites of progesterone showed no effect on ATP-dependent calcium binding (Figure 16). These were (1) 17α-hydroxyprogesterone, a metabolite that is inactive in women except when used in the form of the caproate; (2) 5α-pregnane-3,20-dione or allopregnanedione, which is found in pregnancy urine and is also inactive; and (3)

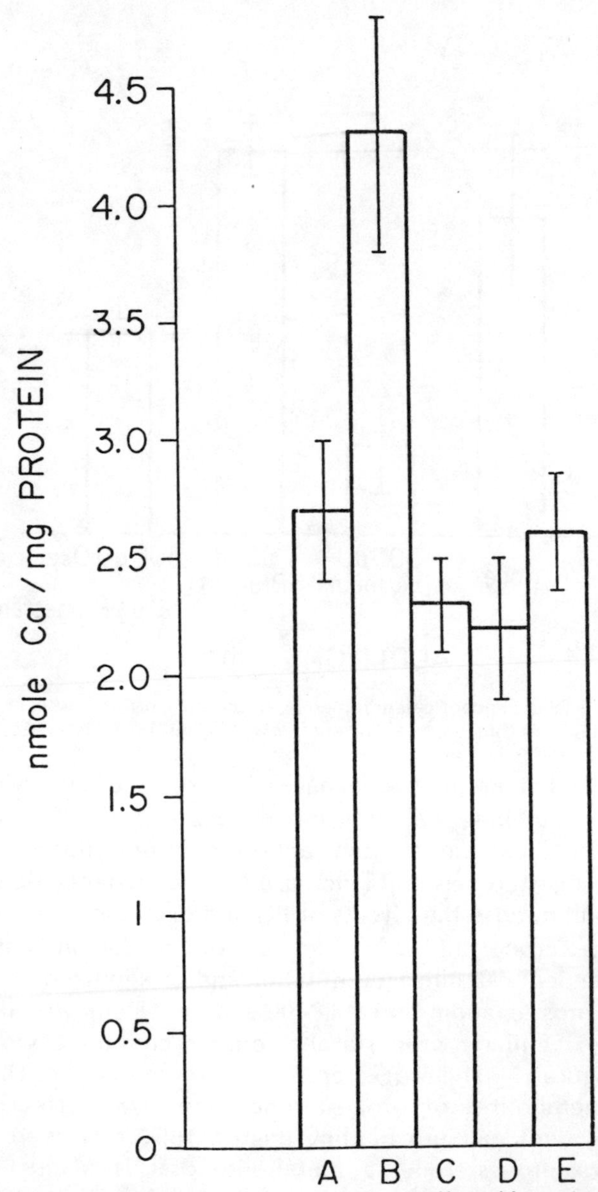

Figure 16. ATP-dependent calcium binding as affected by various additions (50 μg/ml). A: None. B: Progesterone. C: 17α-hydroxyprogesterone. D: Pregnane-3,20-dione. E: 5α/β-Pregnane-3α,20α-diol. From Carsten, M.E. *Gynecol. Invest.* 5:269, 1974.

5β-pregnane-3,20α-diol or pregnanediol, the chief metabolite of progesterone. These findings suggest that the uterine blocking action of progesterone may be mediated through its effect on calcium translocation.

Table 3 summarizes our observations. They suggest that the regulatory effect of prostaglandins or oxytocin on calcium transport may be the basis for the increased contractile force of the uterus observed in labor and perhaps for the onset of labor. The blocking action of progesterone appears to have an opposite effect on ATP-dependent calcium binding and thus antagonizes the actions of prostaglandins and oxytocin on the cellular level.

Table 3
Hormonal Effects on Calcium Translocation

PG and oxytocin inhibit ATP-dependent calcium binding

$PGE_2 > PGF_{2\alpha}$
Third trimester pregnant uterus more sensitive to $PGF_{2\alpha}$ than nonpregnant uterus
Third trimester pregnant uterus much more sensitive to oxytocin than nonpregnant uterus
PG and oxytocin are synergistic

PG and oxytocin release previously bound calcium

$PGE_2 > PGF_{2\alpha}$
$PGF_{1\beta}$ had no effect

Progesterone enhances ATP-dependent calcium binding

Progesterone opposes $PGF_{2\alpha}$ effect
Progesterone opposes oxytocin effect

PHYSIOLOGIC IMPLICATIONS OF HORMONE ACTION

It is well documented that hormones have an initial action at the cell membrane. Excitatory action results in depolarization of the cell membrane with an action potential discharge and influx of inorganic ions.

In addition, there is considerable evidence that the stimulus which makes smooth muscle contract may not be entirely an electrical event mediated by alteration of the membrane potential. It is thought that agents which excite smooth muscle owe at least part of their activity to a direct intracellular effect. Tension can develop in response to the application of various endogenous neurohumoral agents or polypeptides to the external cell membrane, and this tension may not correlate with changes in membrane polarization. This phenomenon is called pharmacomechanical coupling.[11]

It follows (1) that prostaglandins might penetrate the cell membrane. This could then release a second messenger—for example, a cyclic nucleotide—which in turn would react with the SR. (2) The second mode of action would be direct action on the SR. Specific receptor sites for PG have been found in microsomal preparations from the myometrium by Kirton[12] and by us. However, since it is not known whether these binding sites are in the SR or in plasma membrane present accidentally in the preparation, we cannot distinguish between direct PG action on the SR and action on the plasma membrane followed by release of a cyclic nucleotide. (3) A third mode of action is that PG interacts with a calcium-binding mechanism located in the plasma membrane. In that case, the microsomal preparations would have to contain plasma membrane which functions in vivo by pumping calcium out of the cell, and the plasma membrane vesicles must be turned inside out.

There is evidence from muscle bath experiments that cyclic AMP (cAMP) is involved in uterine muscle relaxation.[13] No causal relationship of cAMP to contraction could be established, however.[14] Beta-adrenergic agents, which are thought to act through a cAMP mechanism (such as ritodrine, solbutamol, and tolbutamine), have been successfully used in the prevention of premature labor. However, the relation of ATP-dependent calcium binding to cAMP levels is still unclear.

It is well to keep in mind that even if a change in cAMP were found, this does not necessarily mean that cAMP is an obligatory and/or specific intermediate in the relaxation of the uterus. Therefore, many observations in this direction are presently undergoing further scrutiny. As for prostaglandins, it has not been documented that they act through a cyclic nucleotide mechanism in this system.

CONCLUSIONS

The study of basic biochemical aspects and of the regulatory mechanisms of uterine contractility may lead to a better understanding of physiologic events relating to parturition in which PG is involved. Proper performance of the uterine contractile system is of prime importance in normal pregnancy and parturition. It is conceivable that defects in the cellular calcium transport may be the specific lesion which may cause premature labor, uterine dystocia, or postpartum hemorrhage, and can lead to life-threatening complications or debilitating disease for mother and/or fetus.

In attempts to correct any malfunction, one is faced with the problem that the constituent parts of the contractile system of the uterus are not much different from the same parts in other systems, ie, in organs other than the uterus. Thus, actomyosin or AM-like proteins are not only found in all muscle cells, but are also present in the brain, neurons, platelets, erythrocytes, and in fact in all motile cells. Possibly, a way to reach an understanding of the contractile machinery of the uterus is by using uterine-specific hormones as regulatory agents. At present it appears that prostaglandins are agents of primary importance in this regard.

DISCUSSION

Dr. Work: When you were examining the symbiotic effect of oxytocin and prostaglandins, did you approach it quantitatively? Was the dose of oxytocin held constant, while increasing quantities of PG were added?

Dr. Carsten: No, we performed one short experiment using middle-range concentrations of both agents based on our log dose-response curves aiming at obtaining about a 50% effect of each. I could not speculate on the kinds of variations we would have obtained if we had altered the levels. As to whether or not we might have achieved a plateau effect, this was not assessed specifically because we chose concentrations deliberately to ensure we would not have a maximum effect of either compound. We felt we would be able thereby to determine the effect of the other agent. I can only wonder if this would really be a fruitful line of research to pursue; I would doubt that it would yield any benefit unless there is some great clinical importance in using both agents—oxytocin and PG—in combination.

Dr. Work: It has intriguing possibilities. There are some clinical situations in which we attempt to induce uterine activity but face the frustration of failure because the agent we use cannot achieve the uterotonic effect we seek. From time to time, we wonder if what we observe in $PGF_{2\alpha}$ inductions is not perhaps the result of subtle mechanisms acting on the cellular level. They are undoubtedly more sophisticated than the gross changes we see in terms of the uterine activity response and changes in the cervix. Surely, it would be of considerable practical value if such effects could be modified or controlled by appropriate overlap, admixture, or sequencing of agents. There is a logical basis for our interest. Moreover, there is some reported suggestive clinical evidence that PG sensitizes the uterus to oxytocin. If this proves to be correct, the subject would well be worthwhile investigating further.

Dr. Friedman: What establishes the rhythmicity of the contraction-relaxation cycle on the biochemical level? What is happening inside the cell at different phases of the cycle? Is there a consistent flux back and forth and, if so, what triggers it?

Dr. Carsten: If you are referring to the waveform of the contractile response of the uterus acting as an intact, functioning organ system, we might have to evoke the possibility of a pacemaker site and slow conduction of impulse spreading throughout the uterus. On the cellular level, there is release of calcium triggered either through an electrical event or by a pharmacologic or physiologic agent. The calcium released from cellular stores becomes available to the actomyosin for contraction. As this process proceeds in its course, the ATP runs out. The cell relaxes and the calcium is pumped back into the storage areas or out into the extracellular fluid where it remains until the next impulse comes along.

Dr. Friedman: We all recognize, of course, that there is as yet no substantive proof of a definable pacemaker site or conduction system in the human uterus, although it has been clearly demonstrated in some lower animals. This deserves to be explored in greater depth. On a more relevant issue, you mentioned that the calcium-binding inhibition was greater in the pregnant bovine uterus than in the nonpregnant with reference to $PGF_{2\alpha}$. Do you have comparable data with regard to PGE? Further, was the effect achieved ever maximal? You demonstrated a fine degree of inhibition with oxytocin concentrations of 50 μU/ml in the pregnant bovine uterus, but were you able to attain 100% inhibition with $PGF_{2\alpha}$ when it was used in conjunction with oxytocin? I am wondering whether it is possible to saturate the system and in effect totally inhibit. In addition, again with regard to the additive effects of oxytocin and PG, were you able to assess an index of the level of PG circulating within the cell or, more pertinently, within your microsomal preparations? After all, PG is a rather ubiquitous group of substances and is undoubtedly already present in the cytosol. Were you, therefore, adding critical levels or was it indeed necessary to add critical levels at that point? Finally, did you consider using PG antagonists in order to demonstrate whether the oxytocin effect might not have been manifest by way of a PG mechanism?

Dr. Carsten: A maximum calcium-binding inhibition effect was obtained in the pregnant uterus. I am convinced there was very nearly total inhibition in this preparation. The preexisting level of PG was very low, and I believe we lost some of it in the experiment. We were able to measure it. We have not as yet used any PG antagonists, nor have we studied the effects of PG analogues either.

Dr. Noah: Is it true the more lipophilic a compound is, the less ionophoretic it is?

Dr. Carsten: No, I may have given a wrong impression in this regard. This consideration arose purely because of anticipated experimental difficulties. We needed a solvent that was not water soluble so as to provide us with the required three layers for our study, yet polar enough to get PGE_2 into solution at higher concentrations.

Dr. Hayashi: Would you care to speculate on the clinical observation that PG induction of labor may result in more uterine polysystole, hypertonus, or hypercontractility than oxytocin? If correct, could this relate to different mechanisms of action of these agents?

Dr. Carsten: Muscle tone may somehow be related to the process by which calcium enters the cell, whereas sustained tetanic reactions are thought to be related to the calcium stored within the cell. I fear we are now hypothesizing well beyond our limited knowledge, reaching out from information we have gathered on an essential basic intracellular control mechanism, skipping over numerous undefined steps, to consider a physiologic endpoint, in a clinical setting.

Dr. Friedman: We would like to know the mechanism by which PG may affect contractility and in what way it may differ from oxytocin or from spontaneous contractility. I recognize we just do not have sufficient data at this time to say. However, your data may touch on this matter in a way that may be worth talking about because it may help to distinguish modes of action, particularly as they may affect the relaxation aspect of the contractile cycle. Without dealing with pacemaker and conduction considerations, could we undertake to conjecture that relaxation is perhaps an active process and is not merely the passive result of the contraction phenomenon? If it were active, perhaps a mechanism involving cAMP pertains. Therefore, it is possible that PG does not act by way of the sarcoplasmic reticulum, but through the plasma membrane affecting the calcium pump. Although this may not be correct, I think it is logical and consistent with what you have demonstrated in your microsomal preparations. Oxytocin, on the other hand, may work primarily intracellularly without affecting the plasma membrane to any great extent. If the recovery phase of the contraction cycle involving cAMP has more to do with intracellular and SR activity than with plasma membrane, perhaps we have a means for showing distinct differences in its action on relaxation as opposed to comparable kinds of action on contraction. This is all speculative, of course, but your thoughts would be appreciated.

Dr. Carsten: We are presently involved in trying to separate our preparations further into SR and cell membrane components. This is difficult at best. Harbon and coworkers[15] have shown that epinephrine added to muscle strips increases cAMP levels. By and large, epinephrine relaxes the uterus, so that cAMP is somehow involved in the relaxation process. Moreover, cAMP is also increased when PGE_1 is added. This really does not make sense because PGE_1 contracts the uterus. We must try to determine what the relationship is between PG and cAMP in this system. No consistent relation with cAMP has been uncovered so far, but work is being done along these lines.

You mentioned the possibility that relaxation is an active process. The thought crossed my mind that, if relaxation requires sustained positive action of some kind, an uncontrolled cellular mechanism might result from consumption of whatever the key ingredients are. This concept has an appealing ring, even though we usually think about the process the other way around. We generally consider the resting state as a relaxed condition developing out of the exhaustion of the excitatory phase. From our work, we know that ATP is necessary on a cellular level for an active contraction of the actomyosin system. It is also necessary for relaxation in transport of calcium. It is needed as the energy for translocating calcium to the organelles and for pumping it out of the cell in the relaxation process.

Dr. Seitchik: Is there perhaps a difference in contractile mechanism as related to cAMP according to whether a contraction is spontaneous or evoked? We have been led to believe that cAMP is not involved in the former, but may be in the latter. Perhaps cAMP plays a role in protecting the myocyte from overstimulation. We have all seen hypercontractility result while a constant rate of oxytocin infusion was being given to a gravid patient. Moreover, with no change in dose, the uterus will again reduce its response, diminish its resting pressure and the amplitude, frequency, and duration of contractions. Obviously, the uterus is capable of escaping from overstimulation through some unknown mechanism that may not be involved in the physiology of the contraction.

We should not confuse the mechanics of contraction as relaxation with this issue of calcium transport that raises and lowers calcium concentration in the cell. I am aware of only one series of measurements of intracellular calcium obtained during contraction of a muscle cell, and it was not a smooth muscle cell. The maximum concentration was achieved at the time of maximum rate of rise in the tension. By the time the peak tension was reached, the calcium concentration had returned to its resting state. If this holds true for smooth muscle, the calcium event is over when the muscle reaches full tension. There should be no further changes in calcium concentration during the phase of mechanical relaxation.

Dr. Carsten: Whenever a question is raised about how labor comes about, cAMP is invoked. I fully agree that cAMP has not been conclusively shown to be involved here. Experimental data available to us thus far have had some technical shortcomings, particularly because whole muscle strips were studied. More sophisticated work is currently in progress and may resolve the issue in due course. As to calcium transit, it is very difficult to know what is being measured. During active contraction, the calcium is combined in the actomyosin system and, therefore, would not appear as free calcium. Of course, as soon as actomyosin separates into actin and myosin again, it would be released. The precise movement in time would have to be known in order to judge the significance of a particular measurement.

Dr. Work: Is anything known about the role of the mitochondria and cell nucleus in the contractile process?

Dr. Carsten: The nucleus contains a great deal of calcium. What it does there and whether it has anything at all to do with contraction is unknown. The mitochondria store considerable amounts of calcium. In nonmuscle cells, they are believed to be the main organelles responsible for calcium homeostasis. Muscle contraction is a quick reaction and it appears that the calcium uptake into mitochondria at low concentrations is a rather slow process. Therefore, it is unlikely that mitochondria are important elements involved in the release and uptake of calcium in the contraction-relaxation cycle. However, if it can be shown that calcium can be taken up at a rapid velocity, then we would have to revise our thinking. Meanwhile, the mitochondria appear to be primarily engaged in a storage function, rather than the active contractile process.

REFERENCES

1. Siegman, M.J., and Gordon, A.R. Potentiation of contraction: Effects of calcium and caffeine on active state. *Am. J. Physiol.* 222:1587, 1972.

2. Van Breemen, C., Farinas, B.R., Casteels, R., et al. Factors controlling cytoplasmic Ca^{2+} concentration. *Philos. Trans. R. Soc. Lond.* 265:57, 1973.

3. Devine, C.E., Somlyo, A.V., and Somlyo, A.P. Sarcoplasmic reticulum and excitation-contraction coupling in mammalian smooth muscles. *J. Cell Biol.* 52:690, 1972.

4. Popescu, L.M. Cytochemical study of the intracellular calcium distribution in smooth muscle. In R. Casteels, T. Godfraind, and J.C. Ruegg (Eds.). *Excitation-Contraction Coupling in Smooth Muscle.* New York: Elsevier/North-Holland, Inc., 1977.

5. Somlyo, A.P., Vallieres, J., Garfield, R.E., et al. Calcium compartmentalization in vascular smooth muscle: Electron probe analysis and studies on isolated mitochondria. In N.L. Stephens (Ed.). *The Biochemistry of Smooth Muscle.* Baltimore: University Park Press, 1977.

6. Vinogradow, A., and Scarpa, A. Initial velocities of calcium uptake by rat liver mitochondria. *J. Biol. Chem.* 248:5527, 1973.

7. Carsten, M.E., and Miller, J.D. Effects of prostaglandins and oxytocin on calcium release from uterine microsomal fraction. *J. Biol. Chem.* 252:1576, 1977.

8. Carsten, M.E. Prostaglandins and oxytocin: Their effects on uterine smooth muscle. *Prostaglandins* 5:33, 1974.

9. Carsten, M.E., and Miller, J.D. Comparison of calcium association constants and ionophoretic properties of some prostaglandins and ionophores. *Arch. Biochem. Biophys.* 185:282, 1978.

10. Carsten, M.E. Hormonal regulation of myometrial calcium transport. *Gynecol. Invest.* 5:269, 1974.

11. Somlyo, A.V., and Somlyo, A.P. Electromechanical and pharmacomechanical coupling in vascular smooth muscle. *J. Pharmacol. Exp. Ther.* 159:129, 1968.

12. Kirton, K.T., Spilman, C.H., Wyngarden, L.J., and Kimball, F.A. Prostaglandin E_1 specific binding in human myometrium. *Biol. Reprod.* 31:482, 1975.

13. Triner, L., Nahas, G.G., Vulliemoz, Y., et al. Cyclic AMP and smooth muscle function. *Ann. NY Acad. Sci.* 185:458, 1971.

14. Diamond, J., and Hartle, D.K. Cyclic nucleotide levels during carbachol-induced smooth muscle contractions. *J. Cyclic Nucleotide Res.* 2:179, 1976.

15. Harbon, S., Vesin, M., and Clauser, H. Rôle de prostaglandines dans la regulation de la motilité et de l'activité adenylate cyclase du muscle utérin. *Les Prostaglandines Seminaire Inserm.* Paris: privately printed, 1973, p. 8.

3 Control of Uterine Circulation

William H. Clewell

Just as all nutrients, respiratory gases, and waste products are carried to and from the fetus by the umbilical circulation, they must also be carried to and from the uterus by the uterine circulation. Little is known about the control of this vascular bed under physiologic conditions. A more thorough understanding of the mechanisms controlling uterine circulation would perhaps lead to better understanding of such perinatal problems as fetal asphyxia, intrauterine growth retardation (IUGR), toxemia, and abruptio placentae. Furthermore, experimental models of chronic uterine ischemia will aid our understanding of the mechanisms of IUGR and fetal asphyxia.

In this paper I will review our knowledge of the control of uterine circulation, including the mechanisms of estrogen-induced vasodilatation. I will also describe some preliminary experiments with the reduction of the uterine blood flow in pregnant animals.

UTERINE CIRCULATION IN NONPREGNANT ANIMALS

The sheep is a convenient animal for studies of reproductive physiology. It is by nature a docile animal and adapts easily to the laboratory environment. The size of the animals (60 to 90 kg) makes the surgical preparation of animals for chronic physiologic studies technically reasonable. They are hearty and tolerate surgery well, even procedures involving fetal catheters.

For studies involving uterine circulation they offer several advantages in addition to those mentioned above. More than 90% of the uterine blood flow is carried by the two uterine arteries.[1] Thus, electromagnetic flow measurement using bilateral uterine artery flow transducers will reflect essentially the entire uterine perfusion. Furthermore, there are few functionally significant anastomoses between the two uterine arteries.[2] This is in sharp contrast to the uterine circulation in primates. There are two separate arterial supplies in the primate uterus, the uterine arteries and the ovarian arteries. Depending upon the location of the placenta, the bulk of its perfusion will be supplied by a particular artery or arteries. In the sheep with a singleton pregnancy, the placenta is distributed throughout both horns and thus receives perfusions via both uterine arteries. Manipulations of uterine blood flow can be carried out in one horn, leaving the other to serve as a control.

The initial studies of uterine circulation have been carried out in nonpregnant animals. Animals were chronically prepared with bilateral uterine artery electromagnetic flow transducers and uterine artery catheters (Figure 17). Details of the anesthesia and surgical procedure have been described previously.[2,3]

These animals have been used to study the response of the uterine circulation to a number of naturally occurring and synthetic substances. Of compounds which dilate the uterine vasculature, estrogens have the most dramatic effect. Following a very brief exposure to relatively high concentrations of estrogen, the uterine circulation undergoes a marked and prolonged vasodilatation. Injection of 1 μg of estradiol over one minute into one uterine artery will induce a maximal increase

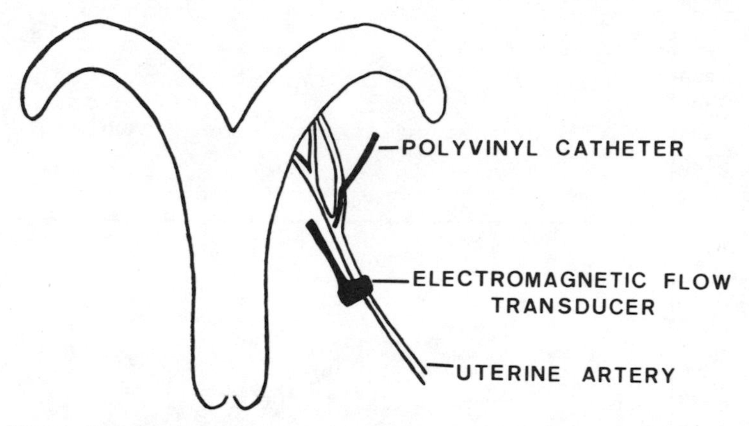

Figure 17. Diagram of surgical preparation. Electromagnetic blood flow transducer around the uterine artery and polyvinyl catheter in a branch of the uterine artery. From Clewell, W.H., et al. *Am. J. Obstet. Gynecol.* 129:384, 1977.

in blood flow in that uterine artery. The time course of this response is characterized by a time lag of 20 to 30 minutes followed by a rapid increase in flow. This vasodilatation peaks at approximately two hours after the injection and then gradually declines. By eight hours after the injection, it has returned to preinjection level (Figure 18). With the injection of 1 μg, this response is strictly unilateral. Only at much higher doses does bilateral vasodilatation occur, indicating a systemic effect.[3]

In an attempt to understand the mechanism of estrogen-induced vasodilatation, a number of vasoactive substances were studied in the uterine circulation. No substance which is a more potent vasodilator in the uterus than estrogen has yet been found. Adenosine and bradykinin will induce maximal responses equal to estrogen.[4] Acetylcholine, which has been proposed as a mediator of estrogen-induced vasodilatation, cannot induce similar maximal blood flows. Furthermore, its effect is completely blocked by atropine, which has no effect on the estrogen response.[4]

Histamine has also been proposed as a mediator of estrogen effects. Even at toxic doses administered by way of the uterine artery, the vasodilatation produced is considerably less than that caused by estrogen. The histamine effect can be

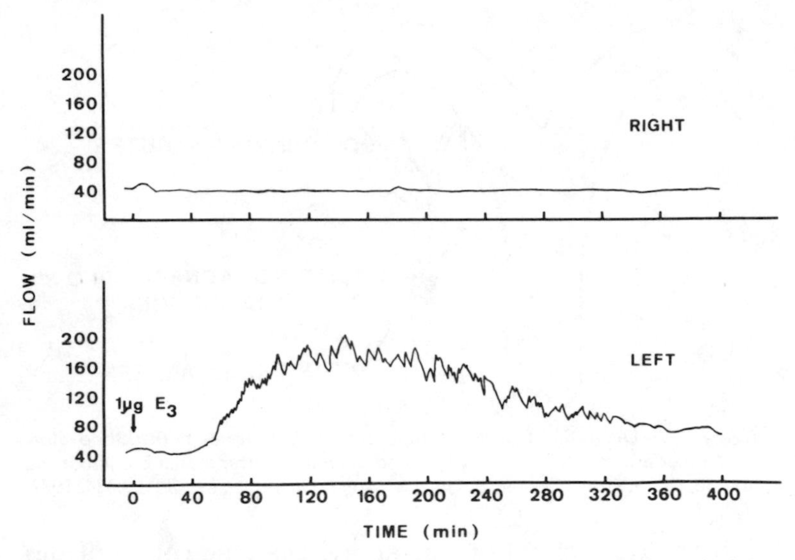

Figure 18. Response of uterine blood flow to 1μg estriol injected into the left uterine artery compared to the response to diluent injected into the right uterine artery. From Clewell, W.H., et al. *Am. J. Obstet. Gynecol.* 129:384, 1977.

completely inhibited by diphenhydramine, which has no effect on the estrogen response.[4]

Beta-adrenergic stimulation has been hypothesized as a mechanism of estrogen-induced vasodilatation. Intraarterial isoproterenol infusion, however, cannot equal the vasodilatation induced by estrogen. The beta-blocker propranolol has no effect on estrogen-induced vasodilatation, whereas it completely inhibits the effects of beta agonists.[4]

Steroid hormones appear to exert their effect on target cells by binding to specific receptors within the cytoplasm. This receptor-steroid complex then moves to the nucleus where it undergoes a confirmational change and binds to the chromatin. The steroid then exerts its effects by initiating the transcription of ribosomal and messenger RNA.[5] It has not been conclusively proven that estrogen-induced vasodilatation requires all the steps involved in this mechanism of action. The observation that the effect is completely blocked by cyclohexamide implies that peptide synthesis is necessary.[2]

Resnik et al. tried to inhibit the response with actinomycin-D and were unsuccessful.[6] Even with local intraarterial infusions of actinomycin-D, it is impossible to inhibit RNA synthesis in vivo completely.

Thus, RNA synthesis is not ruled out as being essential in the response. The 20 to 30 minute lag in the response and the relatively long-term effect are both quite compatible with the proposed mechanism of action. We have also observed that with prolonged exposure to high doses of estrogen, tachyphylaxis can be induced. When this occurs, the organ will continue to show vasodilatation in response to adenosine and bradykinin, but not to estrogen.[7]

The physiologic significance of estrogen-induced vasodilatation remains uncertain. The magnitude of the response is impressive. Peak flows in nonpregnant animals approximate those of midgestation. It seems unlikely that this is merely a pharmacologic phenomenon. With bolus doses, the peak arterial concentrations are quite high (1 γg estradiol injected over one minute leads to brief concentration peaks of approximately 0.05 γg/ml). We have shown, however, that equal degrees of vasodilatation can be achieved with the same total dose injected over 25 minutes. This corresponds to approximately 1.6 ng/ml arterial concentration. We have also shown that with a continuous infusion which produces an arterial concentration of 3 ng/ml, uterine tachyphylaxis to estrogen-induced vasodilatation occurs. In the nonpregnant and pregnant ewe, estrogen concentrations range from 1 to 10 pg/ml. The fetus, however, has estrogen concentrations of 1 to 10 ng/ml.[8] The estrogens in the fetal circulation occur principally as sulfate esters. It is possible that under physiologic conditions the uterine vasculature is exposed to estrogen levels comparable to those in our experiments. Therefore, estrogen may be involved in the physiologic hyperemia of pregnancy.

In late pregnancy, the uterine vasculature appears to be maximally dilated or is at least tachyphylactic to estrogen. No vasoactive substance will induce additional vasodilatation in the near-term sheep uterus.

CONTROL OF CIRCULATION IN PREGNANT ANIMALS

As noted above, the uterine vascular bed of the near-term animal appears to be maximally dilated. Blood flow cannot be increased by estradiol, adenosine, or bradykinin. The vascular bed, however, does not appear to be paralyzed. It responds to vasoconstrictors, such as epinephrine and norepinephrine, with the same sensitivity as in nonpregnant animals.[9] The baseline flow is quite variable over short periods of time (Figure 19). This variability appears to be independent of arterial pressure; it suggests some dynamic control of uterine perfusion. The mechanism of this control is not known. It may operate via vasomotor nerves. The effect of various vasomotor blocking agents on uterine circulation has not been tested.

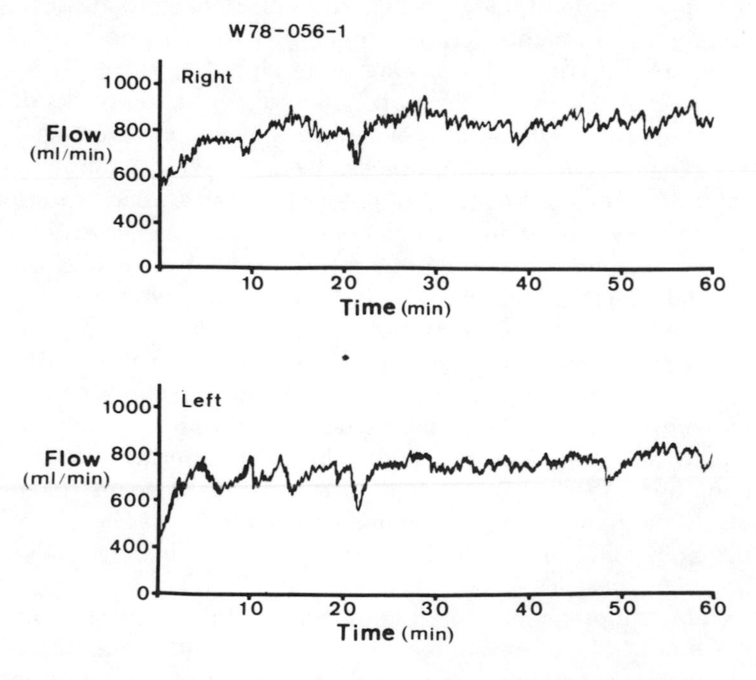

Figure 19. Variability of uterine artery blood flow in a pregnant sheep. Animal connected to flow meter at time zero.

Stress has a striking effect on blood flow in the pregnant animals. Chronically prepared near-term sheep show a dramatic decrease in flow in response to emotional stress. Near-term animals with bilateral uterine flow transducers have a baseline uterine blood flow of approximately 1000 ml/min (combined right and left). For several days after surgery, simply entering the room will cause a 30% to 50% reduction in flow (Figure 19). As the animal becomes more accustomed to the laboratory situation, the magnitude and the duration of the stress responses become less. The most striking thing about this response is that the fetus seems to tolerate it quite well. The fetus routinely survives stress of far greater magnitude in the laboratory (such as preparation for surgery) and in nature (the presence of potential predators). These observations suggest that the uterine circulation is very responsive during pregnancy. Furthermore, the normal fetus exists with an enormous reserve in terms of uterine perfusion.

While the fetus tolerates moderate acute, short-term reduction in uterine blood flow, the effects of prolonged restriction have not been directly studied. Creasy et al. used placental embolization as a model of growth retardation.[10] In these experiments, they embolized the placenta with 15 micron microspheres until mild fetal hypoxia occurred. They did not measure uterine flow in their studies. At sacrifice, they found that one-third of the placental cotyledons were grossly abnormal. This implies that perhaps a 30% reduction in placental perfusion had occurred. The fetuses in these pregnancies suffered definite growth retardation.

This mechanism of reduction of blood flow is physiologically distinct from that produced by vasoconstriction. Figure 20 compares the effect on placental function of placental embolization with that of vasoconstriction. In both cases of flow reduction, the total placental perfusion on the maternal side is reduced by 50%. The model in the figure is for a hypothetical, strictly flow-limited substance (Figure 20 A). Two effects should be noted. First is the change in placental clearance with reduction of blood flow. Clearance is a measure of the efficiency with which the placenta exchanges a

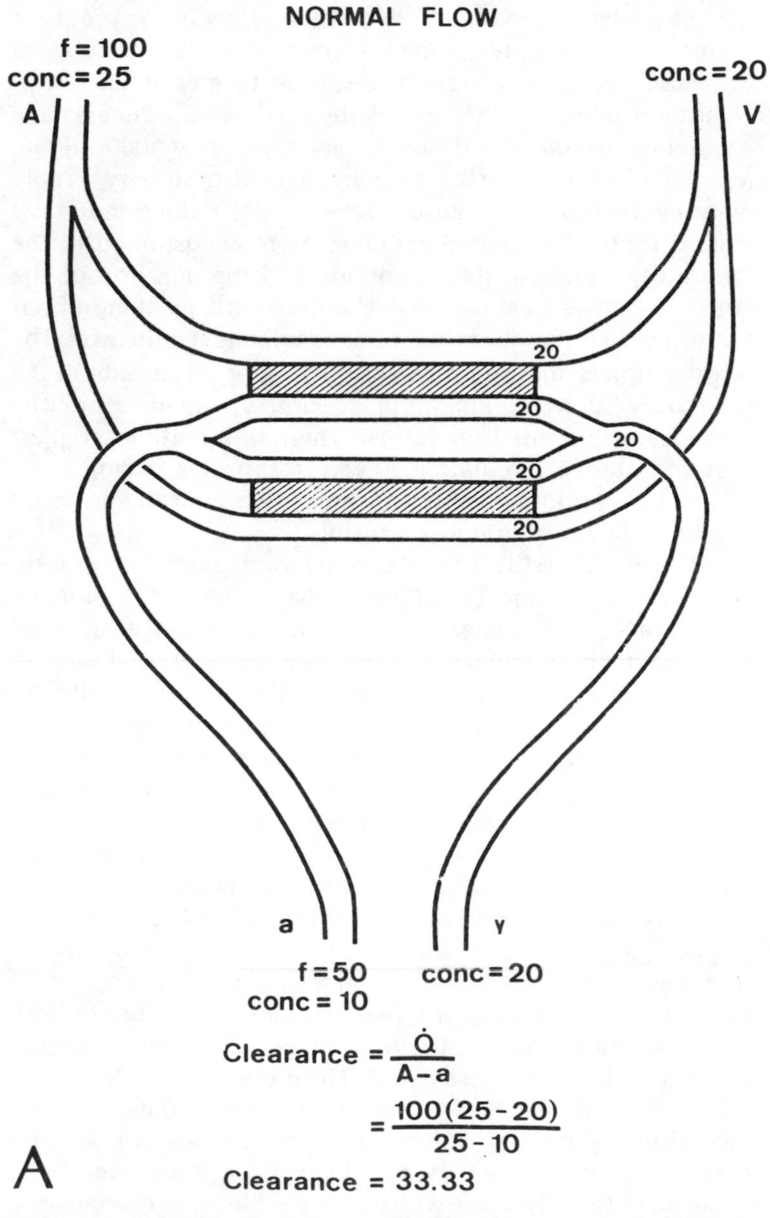

Figure 20. A Model of placental clearance of a purely flow-limited substance. Maternal blood flow is 100, fetal flow is 50. Umbilical arterial concentration is 10, venous is 20. Clearance is 33.33.

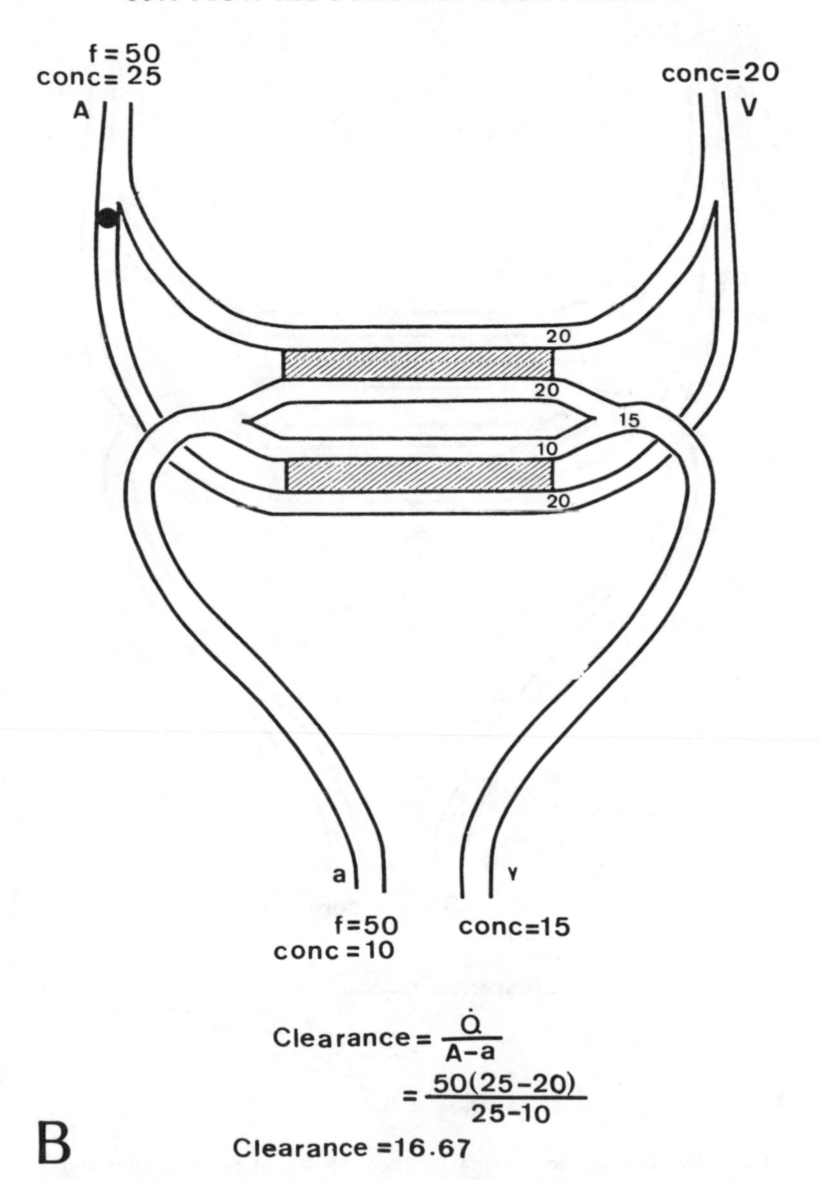

Figure 20. B Effect on placental function of 50% maternal flow reduction by embolization. Maternal blood flow is 50, fetal flow is 50. Umbilical arterial concentration is 10, venous is 15. Clearance is 16.67.

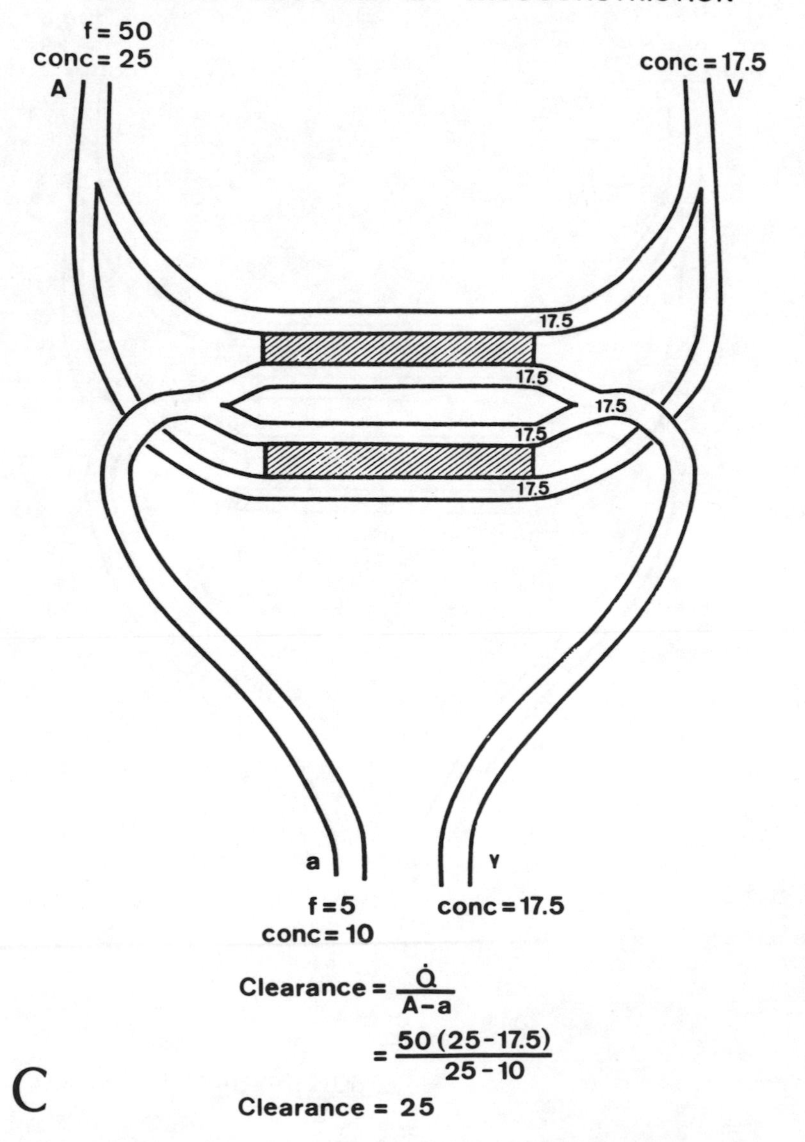

Figure 20. C Effect on placental function of 50% maternal flow reduction by uniform vasoconstriction. Maternal blood flow is 50, fetal flow is 50. Maternal arterial concentration is 25, venous is 17.5. Clearance is 25.

particular substance. As can be seen in the model, embolization (Figure 20 B) results in a much more severe reduction of placental clearance than does vasoconstriction (Figure 20 C). The second feature to note is the reduction of the umbilical venous concentration of our hypothetical flow-limited substance. Again, embolization has a far more severe effect than does vasoconstriction.

Oxygen and carbon dioxide are essentially flow-limited substances in the sheep placenta. If we were to construct a model for membrane-limited substances, the difference between the effect of embolization and that of uniform vasoconstriction would be even more dramatic. Fetal nutrients, such as glucose and amino acids, are handled by the placenta in a membrane-limited fashion.

The clinical circumstance of utero-placental insufficiency may involve elements of both uniform flow restriction and infarction. Therefore, the metabolic consequences of both types of flow reductions must be investigated in order for us to understand the clinical syndrome of intrauterine growth retardation.

CONCLUSIONS

1. The uterine circulation is under dynamic control in both pregnant and nonpregnant animals.

2. Estrogens are the most potent vasodilating agents in this vascular bed. They may be involved in the vasodilatation of pregnancy.

3. The uterine vascular bed is sensitive to catecholamines in both pregnant and nonpregnant states. Psychologic stress induces pronounced uterine vasoconstriction in pregnant animals. This may be mediated by either circulating or local catecholamine release. The fetus tolerates moderately acute, brief reductions in flow quite well.

4. There are at least two different experimental models for utero-placental insufficiency. Fetal growth retardation has been produced in experimental animals by placental embolization. This, however, is physiologically distinct from the effect of generalized uterine ischemia. Both models must be studied before a complete understanding of utero-placental insufficiency and growth retardation can be achieved.

DISCUSSION

Dr. Work: Could you address yourself briefly to the issue of autoregulation of uterine artery flow? This seems to be a most important aspect of your work insofar as it relates to clinical problems.

Dr. Clewell: Fluctuations in flow reflect proportional changes in blood pressure. Artificially varying the perfusion pressure over quite a wide range, however, provides no evidence at all of autoregulation of this system in pregnant animals. This matter is not so clear-cut in nonpregnant animals. Flow rates of very small magnitude, furthermore, give rise to methodologic problems. Electronic flow measurement of small flows is difficult primarily because flow transducers are designed to accommodate observations of large flows. We have considered the possibility of using mechanical occluders to obtain true zero blood flow in order to make more precise measurements of small flows, but then we would be introducing a stress situation. This is something we would like to avoid, because stress blunts response to epinephrine. In fact, stress obliterates the response to estrogen. Therefore, it is very important to avoid stressing these animals in any way. At any rate, it has been clearly shown that there is no autoregulation at high flow rates.

Dr. Friedman: Have you been able to show any inhibition of effect in the pregnant animal preparation? If maximum vasodilatation is the normal state in pregnancy, what happens to the tachyphylaxis to continuous exposure to estrogen that is observed to develop in the nonpregnant animal?

Dr. Clewell: In midpregnancy, prior to the time when uterine blood flow has reached 2 l/min, there is a response, although it is blunted and clearly not so great as in comparable nonpregnant animals. Nearer to term, there is no detectable response. We find no additional vasodilatation in the near-term animal in response to estrogen, even when it is given in huge doses. The uterine vasculature must be considered to be maximally dilated at this time. Interestingly, we have not been able to reverse the catecholamine effect with estrogens. We are unable to dilate an artery with estrogen if it has been constricted by catecholamines. It just does not respond to it.

Dr. Friedman: Some of the observations you have made, particularly as related to nonpregnant preparations and the effect of estradiol on increasing uterine blood flow according to whether given by bolus, divided doses, or continuous infusion, are very reminiscent of some early work done on multicompartment systems. I am referring to work emanating from Plentl's[11] laboratory on the origin and fate of amniotic fluid and the quantitation of hypothetical pathways between mother, fetus, and amniotic fluid compartments by multiple tracer experiments. I cannot help wondering whether your contributions would not be made still more meaningful if a multicompartment system were studied, developing a series of equations to help evolve transfer or clearance rates, perhaps on the basis of a mathematical model.

Dr. Clewell: Undoubtedly, there are multiple compartments at the cellular level, including cytoplasmic and nuclear compartments. We have experimented with different empirical equations, but so far none has given us a clear-cut fit. Obviously, we are looking at just one phenomenon as a response to estrogen within the cytoplasm of some not-yet-identified population of cells within the uterus, rather than to circulating serum or plasma levels. Moreover, such relationships have to be correlated with the events occurring intracellularly, such as those so dramatically demonstrated earlier by Dr. Carsten.

Dr. Friedman: On the subject of clinical application, there is a spectrum of clinical conditions that your animal models parallel. Large portions of a placenta may be affected, say by an occlusive thrombotic process, so that considerable placental blood flow is cut off. This will differ from the condition in which there is a more-or-less uniform overall diminution in placental blood flow, say by a vasculitis or generalized vasospasm. The information that may ultimately derive from your various experimental models, therefore, may prove exceedingly useful, provided we can learn to apply such derivative data to the correct clinical state.

The apparent ability of a fetus to withstand hypoxia or anoxia for long periods of time deserves to be questioned. Over wide ranges of oxygen limitation, no change in fetal oxygen consumption appears to be demonstrable. Could this relate somehow to a mechanism which operates during hypoxia by which there is preferential flow to brain and heart? Clearly, oxygen utilization reflects the overall uptake without taking into consideration the distribution within the organism. If the nonvital organs are not being perfused, the diversion results in less utilization of the limited oxygen supply source.

Dr. Clewell: This mechanism surely pertains, but another is also important, namely, invoking anaerobic metabolism. Although a fetus may indeed divert flow away from skeletal muscle, gut, and kidney to supply brain and myocardium, its overall oxygen consumption must fall if only because less oxygen is available. While aerobic metabolism may support the fetus for a short time, it will not last. Dynamically, there must be both diversion of flow and a change from aerobic to anaerobic metabolism. Alternatively, it is conceivable that the fetus could switch skeletal muscle to anaerobic metabolism, thus producing lactate which in turn could be burned in the liver. Thus, the oxygen consumption in the umbilical vessels (where we measure it) may not change, but utilization could be going down in skeletal muscle and simultaneously going up in the liver. There could be different thresholds in different tissues for switching to anaerobic metabolism. Teleologically, it would be very advantageous to the fetus to shut off oxygen consumption in muscle at a relatively high oxygen content compared to brain and myocardium. These latter vital organs can get by with much lower oxygen contents, but their aerobic needs must still be met. Much work needs to be done along these lines.

Dr. Stys: Our clinical impression is, of course, that reduced uterine blood flow results from increased uterine activity, and vice versa. Did you observe changes in uterine contractility associated with either vasodilatation or blood flow reduction, and was there any difference between pregnant and nonpregnant animals in this regard?

Dr. Clewell: We have not as yet had a nonpregnant animal preparation in which we could measure uterine pressure or tone because of technical constraints. In pregnant animals, however, there is no obvious change in uterine pressure based on measurements made with a single manometer. No sustained long-term change in uterine tone occurred during the ischemic episode, but subtle transitory changes would not have been detectable in our preparation.

Dr. Stys: It is conceivable that the estrogen effect you have shown is mediated through prostaglandins. Could you comment on the supportive evidence for this contention?

Dr. Clewell: Current evidence is based on arteriovenous differences observed in prostaglandin levels which are greater during vasodilatation than at other times, although the differences reported are not very impressive. Infusion of E-series prostaglandins into the uterine artery will yield vasodilatation, but not of the magnitude we have observed here. The evidence, therefore, is only suggestive; it is not conclusive. They are undoubtedly mediators of the response, but our knowledge about them is limited.

Dr. Stys: Were maternal blood pressure and heart rate affected by reducing uterine blood flow in the pregnant animals? Is it possible that fetal factors may be responsible for the lack of response to estriol in the pregnant state? Are other maternal blood vessels affected, specifically in the nonreproductive organs?

Dr. Clewell: We observed no changes in either blood pressure or heart rate in the maternal animal. We looked for such effects for two reasons. First, we wanted to see if we were getting any systemic reaction from catecholamines. Second, we were interested in learning whether or not uterine ischemia would result in maternal hypertension. Over the short periods of our experimental investigations, no effect could be shown.

Shutting off fetal circulation also had no apparent effect. Acute fetal death was produced by air embolization. Uterine blood flow did not change for the next 48 to 72 hours, and then it gradually decreased. Thus, oxygen uptake across the uterine circulation fell abruptly, but uterine blood flow did not.

As to estrogen effect on blood flow in nonreproductive organs, experiments have been done using microsphere injection techniques. Estrogens dilate vessels in the uterus, vagina, and mammary glands, but not those in skeletal muscles. There may be estrogen receptors in responsive vessels, but so far they cannot be demonstrated because we are examining whole uterus or myometrium preparations. If it were possible to look only at the precapillary arterioles, perhaps we would find the answer we seek, but such clean preparations are not yet available.

Dr. Hayashi: How can you explain the observed increase and maintenance of maximal blood flow in the pregnant animal as compared with the nonpregnant one? If estrogen mediates maximal vasodilatation, why does not tachyphylaxis develop? In high primates, the vessels supplying the intervillous space are altered by trophoblastic changes. Do comparable degenerative anatomic changes occur in sheep spiral arterioles? Is there some way to measure differential flow within the uterus as related to distribution to the placental bed?

Dr. Clewell: Frank Greiss[12] suggested that progesterone may be involved. He found a progressive decrease in responsiveness with daily sequential administration of estrogen. Giving progesterone causes the response to return. This suggests one needs progesterone for maintenance of response. In our experiments, we have not seen this decrease in responsiveness with time except in association with continuous high-level estrogen administration. If estrogen is a critical mediator of vasodilatation in pregnancy, perhaps it is acting in a pulsatile manner; that is, the vessels are exposed to only a brief burst of estrogen at any given time and at a much lower concentration. In our studies, 1.5 to 1.6 ng/ml for 25 minutes caused maximal dilatation; above 3 ng/ml yields tachyphylaxis. Perhaps some intermediary level might give different results, but the various doses we tried produced either response or tachyphylaxis. We just do not know if there is some special dosage schedule or fluctuating level that will maintain vasodilatation.

As to the spiral arterioles in sheep, they do not undergo the changes seen in primates. They look like normal unaffected vessels in the placental cotyledons that we have dissected and studied histologically. There is no trophoblastic invasion. The paralysis of the circulation cannot be explained on the basis of destruction of the media by trophoblastic invasion. Sheep are, of course, different from primates, but they are a convenient model for such studies. We can readily distinguish that portion of myometrium overlying placental cotyledons or caruncles from the myometrium between them. Microsurgical techniques are available to study these separately to assess differential effects. They both appear to respond about the same to estrogens and to catecholamines. Although there is a slight preferential vasodilatation in the placental part of the endometrium to estrogens, the difference is small.

REFERENCES

1. Rosenfeld, C.R., Killam, A.P., Battaglia, F.C., et al. Effect of estradiol-17β on the magnitude and distribution of uterine blood flow in nonpregnant, oophorectomized ewes. *Pediat. Res.* 7:139, 1973.
2. Killam, A.P., Rosenfeld, C.R., Battaglia, F.C., et al. Effect of estrogens on the uterine blood flow of oophorectomized ewes. *Am. J. Obstet. Gynecol.* 115:1045, 1973.
3. Clewell, W.H., Carson, B.A., and Meschia, G. Comparison of uterotrophic and vascular effects of estradiol-17β and estriol in the mature organism. *Am. J. Obstet. Gynecol.* 129:384, 1977.
4. Resnik, R., Killam, A.P., Barton, M.D., et al. The effect of various vasoactive compounds upon the uterine vascular bed. *Am. J. Obstet. Gynecol.* 125:201, 1976.
5. Chan, L., and O'Malley, B.W. Mechanism of action of the sex steroid hormones. *N. Engl. J. Med.* 294:1322, 1372, 1430, 1976.
6. Resnik, R. Battaglia, F.C., Makowski, E.L., and Meschia, G. The effect of actinomycin-D on estrogen-induced uterine blood flow. *Am. J. Obstet. Gynecol.* 122:273, 1975.
7. Clewell, W.H., Stys, S.J., and Meschia, G. Stimulus summation and tachyphylaxis in estrogen response. Society for Gynecologic Investigation, 24th Annual Meeting, Tucson, Ariz., March 23-25, 1977. *Abstract.*
8. Ferguson, F.A., and Cox, R.I. Hormones. In M.H. Blunt (Ed.). *The Blood of Sheep, Composition and Function.* New York: Springer-Verlag, 1975.

9. Barton, M.D., Killam, A.P., and Meschia, G. Response of ovine uterine blood flow to epinephrine and norepinephrine. *Proc. Soc. Exp. Biol. Med.* 145:996, 1974.

10. Creasy, R.K., Barrett, C.T., DeSwiet, M., et al. Experimental intrauterine growth retardation in the sheep. *Am. J. Obstet. Gynecol.* 112:566, 1972.

11. Plentl, A.A. The dynamics of the amniotic fluid. *Ann. NY Acad. Sci.* 75:746, 1959.

12. Greiss, F.C., Jr., and Anderson, S.G. Effect of ovarian hormones on the uterine vascular bed. *Am. J. Obstet. Gynecol.* 107:829, 1970.

4 Changes in the Cervix at Parturition*

Stanley J. Stys

The role of the cervix during pregnancy and parturition as a functional component of the uterus has received relatively little attention from investigators. Perhaps this is because the cervix has been viewed as a passive sphincter which opens only as a result of strong, rhythmic contractions of the muscular uterine fundus. Nevertheless, evidence that has accumulated over the past 30 years clearly defines an active role for the cervix during parturition. In fact, in humans and in other species, expulsion of the fetus by uterine contractile forces is probably not possible before the cervix undergoes intrinsic changes in its physical properties.

The purpose of this paper is twofold. First, it is a review of a representative group of papers which describe the histologic, biochemical and physical changes in the cervix during

*Some of the data have previously been published in *American Journal of Obstetrics & Gynecology* 130:414-418, 1978.

pregnancy and parturition and the effects of potential mediators of these changes on the cervix. Second, it presents physiologic data documenting changes in the physical properties of the cervix at parturition in a new chronically-instrumented animal model.

REVIEW OF THE LITERATURE

Basic Histologic and Biochemical Changes

In 1947, Danforth[1] reported the results of a histologic study of 12 pregnant and 46 nonpregnant uteri. He concluded that the nonpregnant cervix is predominantly fibrous connective tissue with only 15% smooth muscle. He also determined that the anatomic transition from the fibrous cervix to the muscular lower uterus is abrupt. The isthmus of the uterus is composed primarily of smooth muscle with transitional epithelium. In early pregnancy, the cervix does not change significantly in length. The isthmic portion, however, does elongate in the third month of pregnancy. As the products of conception enlarge, the isthmus unfolds to accommodate them. This unfolding is limited by the fibrous cervix.

Danforth's early work was criticized by several investigators who contended that the cervix was not predominantly fibrous in nature. This conclusion was based on a physiologic study which indicated that the cervix was capable of independent contractility in vivo; moreover, a histologic study indicated that the outer portion of the cervical stroma was muscular in nature. In 1954, Danforth[2] published additional work as a rebuttal to the intervening studies. In total, he examined 104 uteri and reaffirmed his earlier impression that the cervix was composed primarily of fibrous connective tissue. The smooth muscle in the cervix consists of isolated, attenuated strands variable in amount from cervix to cervix. Danforth also studied ten cervical and uterine strips in vitro and found that the cervical tissue showed far less contractility.

Danforth and coworkers[2] were intrigued by the marked differences in consistency of the cervix of nonpregnant women, pregnant women who have experienced no effacement or dilatation, and women at delivery. In 1960, they published a report comparing these three groups.[3] Collagen was determined to be the major connective tissue component of the cervix. During pregnancy, collagen fibers were described as enlarged and swollen, but the integrity of the fiber bundles did not appear to be disturbed. After labor, however, the component fibrils of collagen were found to be dissociated from one another. The reticulum of the cervix was more prominent in the pregnant cervix compared to the nonpregnant, but showed little change after labor. The hydroxyproline percentage of the dry weight was less in the postlabor cervix than in the nonpregnant cervix, indicating a decrease in collagen concentration. Danforth and coworkers concluded that fundamental changes occur in the ground substance at parturition rather than in collagen itself. This modification of ground substance in the cervix would permit dissociation rather than dissolution of collagen fibers during the process of effacement and dilatation.

In 1968, Bryant and coworkers[4] reported their study of 108 pregnant rats. Histologic analyses were correlated with biochemical determinations of hydroxyproline, hexosamine, galactosamine, glucosamine, and water throughout pregnancy, during parturition, and postpartum. Gradual changes were noted in the cervix throughout gestation, with a marked change at parturition. In the postpartum period there was a rapid return to the nonpregnant state. The authors' conclusions were that the rapid increase in cervical hexosamine and water prepartum produces an imbalance in the cohesive and dispersive forces interacting between collagen structural units and that this imbalance results in longitudinal cleavage of the collagen units.

In 1974, Danforth and coworkers[5] reported the results of their study of the effects of pregnancy and labor on the collagen, glycoproteins and glycosaminoglycans of the human cervix. Biopsy specimens of ten nonpregnant women and twelve pregnant women at delivery were used in the study. In comparison to the nonpregnant cervix, the cervix after delivery showed slight increases in water, a marked decline in collagen and glycoprotein, and a marked increase in glycosaminoglycans, the polysaccharide elements of the extracellular matrix of connective tissue. They concluded that collagen fibers are not merely loosened, as they had previously proposed, but that significant collagen destruction occurs by the time women deliver. In addition to the collagen destruction, dramatic changes occur in the composition of ground substance. They concluded, therefore, that cervical dilatation is not a passive process, as has been conjectured by other investigators.

Other investigators have corroborated Danforth's more recent conclusions about the destruction of collagen. In 1978, Kleissl and coworkers[6] reported their study comparing the nonpregnant and intrapartum cervix. Both the acid-soluble fraction and the insoluble fractions of collagen were studied. In the acetic acid-soluble fraction, no differences were noted between nonpregnant and intrapartum specimens in the hydroxyproline/total protein ratio. This ratio is an index of the collagen present. Marked differences, however, were noted in the electrophoretic pattern of the acid-soluble fraction, indicating a marked increase in collagen breakdown products in the postdelivery specimens. Analysis of the insoluble fraction revealed that the hydroxyproline/total protein ratio decreased significantly in the intrapartum group as compared to the nonpregnant group. Thus, this group of investigators concluded that a significant degradation of collagen occurs late in pregnancy or at the time of parturition.

Evidence that changes in the cervical ground substance occur during pregnancy has also been growing. Golichowski,[7] in 1978, reported a study of the changes in glycosaminoglycans in pregnant rats. For the first 15 days of pregnancy, little change was noted compared to nonpregnant specimens. From day 15 through day 21 of gestation, however, marked increases were noted in cervical weight, water content, and the amounts of sulfated hexosamine and uronic acid. Analysis by paper chromatography indicated a large increase in keratan sulfate in the last part of pregnancy. Since dermatan sulfate binds tightly to collagen, whereas keratan sulfate does not bind at all, the increase in keratan sulfate may help to explain the cervical softening that occurs prior to parturition.

The studies described above are representative of investigations carried out over the last 30 years on the histologic and biochemical changes taking place during pregnancy and parturition in cervical tissue of both human and animal subjects. As a group, they indicate that there are subtle histologic changes which correlate with changes in collagen content and ground substance. Nevertheless, the precise relationship between these histologic and biochemical changes of the cervix and the dramatic change in the physical properties of cervical tissue, which allow expulsion of the fetus, still remain unclear. Indeed, the fact that many of the biochemical changes of the cervix appear to occur gradually throughout pregnancy does not correlate well with observations that changes in the physical properties of the cervix can be rather abrupt, occurring in some species in a matter of hours.

Humoral Compounds as Part of the Control Mechanism

The papers we have reviewed resulted from attempts to describe the basic histologic and biochemical changes which occur in the cervix during pregnancy and parturition. The approach of a number of other investigators has been to attempt to identify humoral compounds which are part of the control mechanism of these cervical changes. Relaxin is one such humoral compound which plays a role at parturition in a number of animal species. In 1953, Frieden and Hisaw[8] summarized much of the available information regarding relaxin. At that time, relaxin was measured by biological assay and was found to be present in a number of mammalian species. It was found that relaxin administration to estrogen-primed, ovariectomized, nonpregnant guinea pigs led to changes in the collagen and ground substance of the guinea pig symphysis pubis which were similar to changes which occur in cervical tissue of rats and in humans at parturition. Similar changes could be elicited in mice with administration of relaxin.

Interest in relaxin has grown in recent years with the development of a radioimmunoassay for relaxin. In 1976, O'Byrne and coworkers[9] measured relaxin by radioimmunoassay in pregnant hamsters. During the first seven days of gestation in pregnant hamsters relaxin levels are undetectable. From day 7 through day 15 (the day of parturition), there is a gradual increase in relaxin levels. This increase in relaxin during the last week of pregnancy in pregnant hamsters correlates well with the gradual cervical dilatation which occurs at the same time. Relaxin is also known to have a role in parturition in the pregnant pig.

Sherwood and coworkers[10,11,12] have reported a number of studies using radioimmunoassay techniques for measurement of relaxin. In 1975, they reported the results of peripheral plasma levels of relaxin measured throughout pregnancy in pigs.[10] Relaxin levels were low during the first 100 days of gestation, being approximately 2 ng/ml. There was a gradual increase during the last two weeks before parturition to mean levels of 12 ng/ml. In the last two days before parturition, there was a sharp increase in peripheral relaxin levels to a peak of 146 ng/ml. Within hours after delivery, there was a rapid fall to levels of only 1 ng/ml.

In 1976, Sherwood and coworkers studied the effect of prostaglandin $F_{2\alpha}$($PGF_{2\alpha}$) on peripheral relaxin levels.[11] Two days before normal parturition, on day 112, Sherwood injected the sows with 10 mg of $PGF_{2\alpha}$. Within 45 minutes, there was an increase in peripheral relaxin levels to 13 ng/ml. Parturition was also induced by this process. In 1978, this same team reported the effect of serial progesterone injections in pregnant sows from day 110 to day 113.[12] These injections of progesterone delayed parturition by two days in these animals. However, the progesterone treatment did not delay the increase in relaxin seen two days prior to normal parturition, nor did it delay the onset of lactation. Unfortunately, the status of the cervix during the experiment was not documented.

Estrogen has also been related to cervical changes at parturition. In 1965, Pinto and coworkers[13] reported the results of a study in which estradiol-17β was administered to women at term. They noted a moderate oxytocic effect and also cervical ripening within four to eight hours after administration of the estradiol. They also performed a controlled histologic study of 20 patients and found that the estradiol led to increased cervical edema, vascularity, and basal epithelial vacuolization.

Liggins and coworkers,[14] while studying the effects of stilbestrol on parturition in sheep, made some intriguing observations on the cervix. Eleven sheep were injected with stilbestrol, 20 mg subcutaneously, between day 108 and day 142 of gestation. Uterine contractile sensitivity to oxytocin was measured at 12-hour intervals after the administration of the stilbestrol. At 12 hours, in all eleven animals, the sensitivity to oxytocin had decreased to 10% of the preinjection level. Spontaneous uterine activity occurred in 12 hours in some of the animals and by 24 hours in all of the animals. In nine of the eleven ewes, the cervix did not dilate despite continued uterine activity. In two of the eleven ewes, both of which were beyond 135 days of gestation, normal parturition and delivery occurred within 40 hours after the stilbestrol injection.

Hindson and coworkers[15] in 1967 demonstrated similar results with stilbestrol used to induce uterine contractions in sheep. In their study, the ewes which were beyond 135 days usually delivered, while those less than 135 days did not deliver.

In recent years, prostaglandins have been widely studied in relationship to many physiologic processes, including parturition and dilatation of the cervix. There are numerous studies which indicate increased levels of various prostaglandins at various sites in late pregnancy and during and after parturition. A number of studies have dealt with the effect of prostaglandins on the cervix in particular. In 1970, Najak and coworkers[16] measured isotonic and isometric contractility of isolated nonpregnant cervical strips. They found that prostaglandin E_2 (PGE_2) caused relaxation of the cervical strips. In 1973, Liggins and coworkers[14] reported that $PGF_{2\alpha}$ increased at parturition in sheep in the hours prior to parturition.

In 1975, Dingfelder and coworkers[17] inserted vaginal suppositories containing $PGF_{2\alpha}$ into patients about to have induced abortions and noted a greatly reduced cervical resistance in these patients. In 1975, Weiss and coworkers[18] administered oral PGE_2 to multiparous patients at term with unripe cervix and noticed a significant improvement of the Bishop score. In 1976, Conrad and Ueland[19] measured the stretch modulus of human cervical biopsy material. They found that the stretch modulus was significantly decreased in patients who had had induction with PGE_2 compared to spontaneous laboring patients or nonpregnant patients. In 1976, MacKenzie[20] performed in vivo measurements of cervical pressure in the midtrimester of pregnancy. He noted that PGE_2, $PGF_{2\alpha}$, and oxytocin all had nonspecific effects on cervical pressure, while ergometrine caused contractions of the cervix. In 1976, Fitzpatrick[21] administered $PGF_{2\alpha}$ to pregnant ewes and found that within 48 hours many had a floppy cervix. However, less than half showed any change in their cervix. In 1977, Calder and coworkers[22] noted that extraamniotic treatment with PGE_2 of primigravid patients at term improved the cervical score and led to a 25% reduction in the length of induced labor.

PHYSIOLOGIC DATA IN A SHEEP MODEL

The studies we have reviewed suggest a role for relaxin, estrogens, and several prostaglandins in the control of the changes in the physical properties of the cervix which occur at parturition. The controlling mechanisms of this process, however, still need further definition. The basic histologic and biochemical changes in the cervix at parturition also need further elaboration. Nevertheless, there can be little doubt that the cervix is not a passive sphincter merely overcome by the forces that the uterine musculature generates to expel the fetus.

Although the reviewed papers have contributed greatly to our understanding of the role of the cervix at parturition, there appears to be a need for a model in which dynamic changes in the physical properties of the cervix could be documented during spontaneous parturition or during manipulation of parturitional events with humoral agents. Such a model would also allow correlation of biochemical and histologic parameters with the physical status of the cervix. The purpose of the study to be presented was to establish such a model for investigations of this type.

The sheep was chosen as the experimental animal for this study because extensive data on parturitional changes have been accumulated for this animal and because of its functional anatomy. In pregnancy, the sheep cervix is 10 to 12 cm in length and 1 to 2 cm in outer diameter. Moreover, although the sheep cervix remains rigid until a few hours before delivery, uterine contractions of only 10 to 15 torr overcome the resistance to dilatation of a cervix that is four times as long as the human cervix.

The surgical procedure performed on the sheep in the study is illustrated in Figure 21. To measure the compliance of the sheep cervix, a balloon of high compliance is fixed within the proximal end of the cervical canal by a purse-string suture at the internal os. The suture also serves to isolate the cervix from the uterus mechanically. The balloon is at the center of a thick-walled catheter and is designed to contact a 2 cm segment of cervix when inflated. One end leads distally through the cervix and vagina to a pressure transducer. The other end

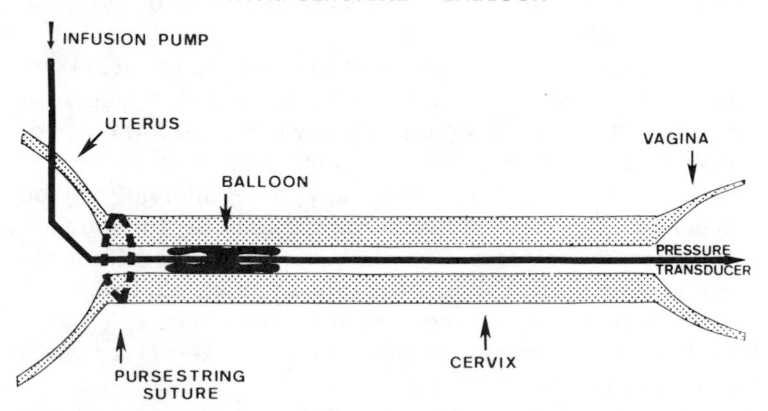

Figure 21. Schematic drawing of position of the intracervical balloon catheter within the cervix of the pregnant ewe. From Stys, S. *Am. J. Obstet. Gynecol.* 130:414, 1978.

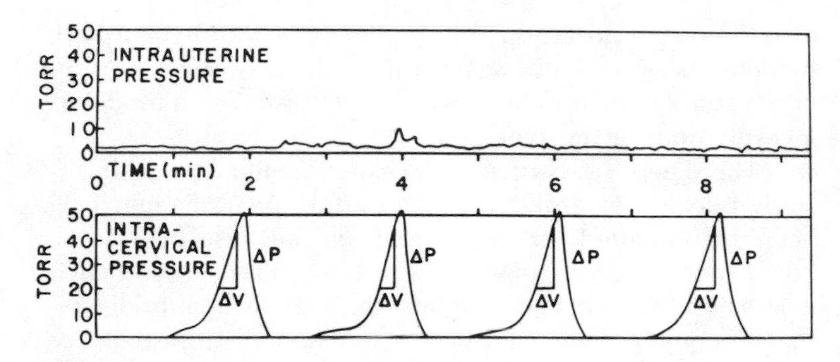

Figure 22. Intrauterine pressure (upper) and intracervical pressure (lower) tracings versus time. Typical pressure-volume curves generated during cervical compliance measurements are demonstrated. Infusion rate was 6.0 ml/min; withdrawal rate was 24.1 ml/min. ΔP refers to pressure change occurring as the volume changed, ΔV. From Stys, S. *Am. J. Obstet. Gynecol.* 130:414, 1978.

leads proximally through the internal cervical os, into the lower uterine segment, then through the uterine and abdominal wall to a constant-rate infusion pump.

Intrauterine pressure is measured simultaneously by a balloon catheter within the uterine cavity. The surgical procedure also includes the placement of an infusion catheter within the fetal femoral vein. Several measurements of cervical compliance are made daily until parturition. Intrauterine and intracervical pressures are recorded continuously in the interim periods.

Representative raw data used to calculate cervical compliance are shown in Figure 22. Intrauterine and intracervical pressures are measured simultaneously over a 50 torr range of pressure. Because the infusion is administered at a constant rate, the volume infused over any time interval can be calculated. As water is infused into the balloon, the intracervical pressure increases. Compliance is calculated from the linear portion of the curve as the ratio of change in volume to change in pressure. The mean of the compliance calculated from four or five pressure-volume curves is taken as the value for cervical compliance for that time.

Nine animals were studied initially; six of them had parturition induced with a fetal infusion of dexamethasone. In three animals with dexamethasone-induced parturition,

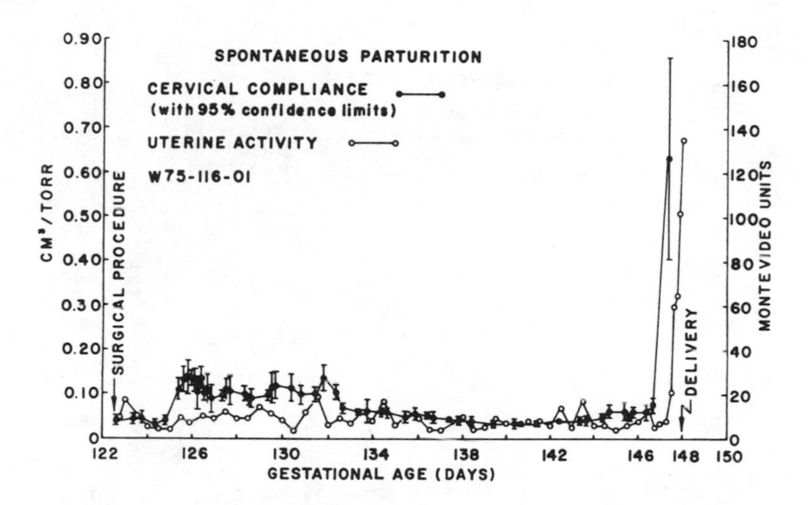

Figure 23. Cervical compliance and uterine activity versus time as gestation advanced for a ewe with spontaneous parturition.

uterine contractions were inhibited with daily injections of progesterone. Three ewes were allowed to undergo spontaneous parturition.

The relationship of cervical compliance and uterine activity versus time in one of the animals experiencing spontaneous parturition is illustrated in Figure 23. The other two animals in this group showed similar patterns. The uterus was quiescent until 12 hours prior to delivery. Two changes in cervical compliance were noted during the study period. Forty-eight hours after surgery, cervical compliance increased threefold and remained elevated for one week, with a gradual return to baseline values. This prolonged increase in cervical compliance demonstrates a physiologic change probably related to surgical stress. It was noted in four of the nine animals in the study. Approximately 24 hours prior to delivery, the compliance of the cervix increased tenfold. This change in compliance preceded the increase of uterine activity characteristic of labor by several hours. Further measurements of cervical compliance could not be made after the abrupt increase noted because of the plastic quality of the cervix after this point.

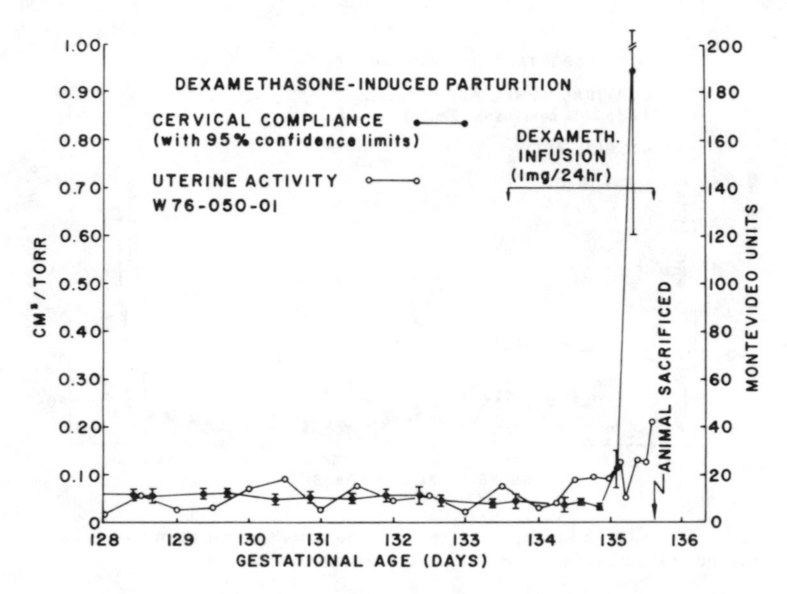

Figure 24. Cervical compliance and uterine activity versus time in gestation for a ewe with dexamethasone-induced parturition.

The relationship of cervical compliance and uterine activity, for an animal with parturition induced with a fetal infusion of dexamethasone (1 mg/24 hours), is illustrated in Figure 24. These data are similar to the data of the other animals treated in the same manner. The surgical procedure for the animal whose data are shown was carried out on day 119 of gestation. The data illustrated encompass only the last eight days of the experiment.

Forty hours after the initiation of the fetal dexamethasone infusion, cervical compliance increased fifteenfold. Uterine activity consistent with early labor began several hours after this dramatic change in cervical compliance. The time relationship between the initiation of the fetal dexamethasone infusion and the onset of labor was consistent with the data reported by Liggins and coworkers[14] for dexamethasone-induced parturition in sheep. This animal was sacrificed shortly after the onset of uterine contractions and confirmation of the plastic, compliant quality of the cervix was made by inspection.

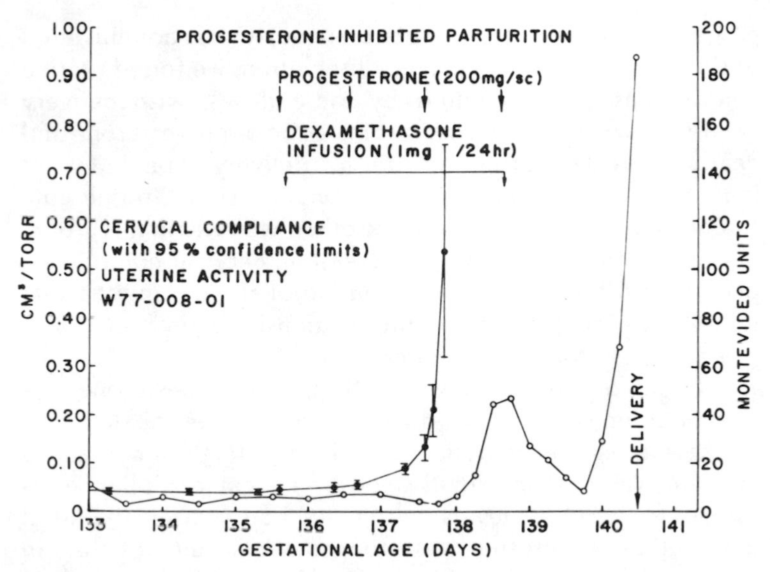

Figure 25. Cervical compliance and uterine activity versus gestational age for a ewe with progesterone-inhibited parturition.

Liggins and coworkers[14] have demonstrated that a daily supplementation of progesterone-in-oil (200 mg subcutaneously) to the ewe will maintain maternal plasma progesterone concentrations and inhibit the onset of uterine contractions, in spite of dexamethasone infusion to the fetus. Lower doses of progesterone will maintain plasma progesterone levels in the ewe but will not inhibit uterine contractions. Curiously, Liggins and coworkers comment that the cervix failed to dilate in this latter group of animals despite adequate uterine contractions.

Intrigued by these data, we performed an experiment to determine whether progesterone administration in amounts sufficient to block uterine activity would also block the increase in cervical compliance in ewes whose fetuses were infused with dexamethasone. Figure 25 illustrates the findings in one of the three animals in this study group. This ewe was prepared on day 130 of gestation, but only the last eight days of the experiment are illustrated. During the 72 hours of dexamethasone infusion, a daily supplementation of progesterone-in-oil (200 mg subcutaneously) was administered to the ewe. Confirming Liggins' observation, we found uterine contractions were inhibited by these doses, with delivery occurring two days after the last injection of progesterone and nearly three days after the time of delivery expected after induction with a fetal dexamethasone infusion. Uterine contractions were also blocked in the other two ewes in this group, but in all animals the abrupt increase in cervical compliance occurred 48 hours after the initiation of the dexamethasone infusion, yielding the same time relationship seen in ewes not given progesterone supplementation.

In one of the three ewes in this group, progesterone supplementation was continued for three days after the dramatic increase in cervical compliance while the fetal dexamethasone infusion was stopped. In this ewe, cervical compliance returned to baseline levels within 48 hours after the fetal dexamethasone infusion was stopped. This indicates that, in the ewe, the cervix is capable of returning to its usual rigid consistency almost as abruptly as it is able to soften in preparation for dilatation. When the fetal dexamethasone infusion was reinstituted seven days later without progesterone supplementation to the ewe, there was a marked increase in cervical com-

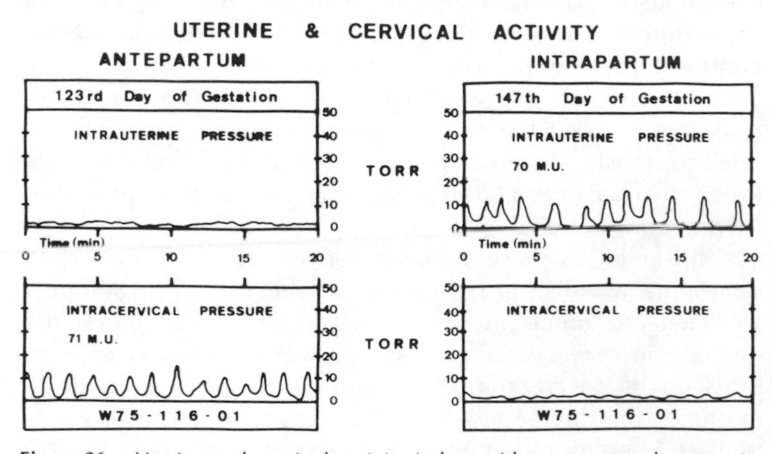

Figure 26. Uterine and cervical activity in late midpregnancy and at term in labor. Typical cervical contractions of the antepartum state and uterine contractions of the intrapartum state are demonstrated. From Stys, S. *Am. J. Obstet. Gynecol.* 130:414, 1978.

pliance concurrent with the initiation of uterine contractions.

Continuous measurements of both intrauterine and intracervical pressure were made throughout the study periods of all ewes studied. Figure 26, which shows raw data, demonstrates the spontaneous uterine and cervical contractions in a ewe which experienced spontaneous parturition. During the antepartum period, the uterus was quiescent, while the cervix contracted rhythmically. During labor, the uterus contracted rhythmically while the cervix was quiescent. Significant cervical contractions were noted in all nine animals in the study.

Figure 27 illustrates uterine and cervical activity versus time during the ewe's entire study period for the same ewe whose contractile pattern is shown in Figure 26. The intensity and frequency of cervical contractions were quite variable over short periods of time, but cervical contractions were common, generally decreasing in amplitude and frequency with the approach of parturition. Consequently, there was a decrease in cervical activity with the approach of parturition. Uterine activity, on the other hand, was minimal prior to the onset of labor.

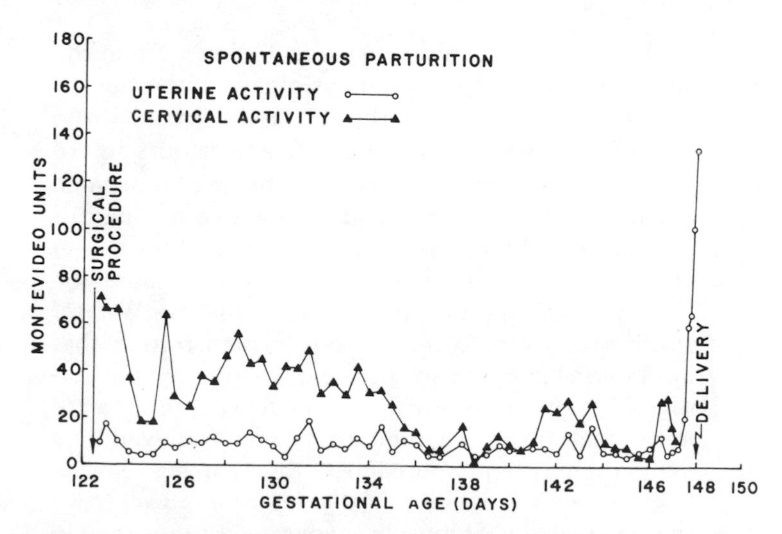

Figure 27. Uterine and cervical contractile activity versus gestational time for a ewe with spontaneous parturition.

CONCLUSION

The purpose of this study was to establish a model to investigate the dynamic changes in the physical properties of the cervix at parturition and the humoral mechanisms which control these changes. The animal model developed can be used to accomplish many of these goals. The data presented provide evidence that the compliance of the cervix increases abruptly during spontaneous and induced parturition in the sheep and that this change in the cervix is independent of uterine contractile activity. In addition, the data indicate that progesterone supplementation to the ewe during induced parturition can inhibit uterine contractile activity but not changes in cervical compliance. It is hoped that further investigations using this model will provide information on the controlling mechanisms of these changes in cervical compliance and on the relationship between the physical, biochemical, and histologic changes in the cervix at parturition.

DISCUSSION

Dr. Friedman: I am sure we will all agree that the anatomy and perhaps the physiology of the human cervix are not the same as that of the sheep cervix. The cervix in the ewe remains rigid until a few hours before labor begins, whereas cervical ripening in women occurs in a more orderly and progressive manner for several weeks before term. Is it possible that the model chosen for study here is inappropriate because the findings may not be applicable to the human? Of specific concern to me is your demonstration that intrauterine pressure and cervical pressure are not correlated in the sheep; further, you showed an increase in cervical pressure early in pregnancy followed by a diminution as term approached. Recognizing that the human cervix contains relatively little muscle, we should expect what muscle is contained to respond in about the same way as the main bulk of myometrium responds to exogenous and endogenous factors. Is the basis for your unexpected findings merely the choice of animal model or is it perhaps some technical problem as well? If the capacity and dimension of the sheep's cervical canal changes with advancing pregnancy, would not your relative measurements of compliance also be altered? The spontaneous contractility seen early in pregnancy is rather an impressive finding. Does its diminution with time reflect the technique of measurement rather than a physiologic change?

Dr. Stys: The cervix of the sheep does tend to hypertrophy somewhat during pregnancy but the canal remains fairly constant until near parturition. More fluid is needed to fill the balloon, indicating that the cervix has dilated. Changes in volume occur before any change is seen in the pressure. The changes in compliance near parturition are quite dramatic in magnitude. It is certainly possible for the exact measurements to be distorted to some extent by dilatation of the canal itself.

The presence of the balloon in the cervical canal may also act as an irritant to some extent, thereby serving to cause some of the contractions that we observed early in pregnancy. The trend in contractility we encountered was clear-cut. The initial effect may be the result of the balloon having just been inserted; subsequent reduction in contractility might just reflect the cervix becoming accustomed to the balloon insertion over the course of a few weeks. There is a good deal of day-to-day variability. The cervix may contract vigorously for six to eight or even twelve hours, then quiet down to a very low level of activity for a few hours, when it may resume more vigorous activity again.

The ripening event in the sheep occurs in a very narrow time frame. This is very different from the human. We have all seen women who efface and dilate their cervix to 3 or 4 cm without entering labor for as long as three to four weeks; others go into labor with a very firm, rigid cervix, and the process of effacement and dilatation occurs over a period of hours in the course of labor. There is much more variability in this regard in the human than in the sheep.

Nevertheless, some basic mechanisms of cervical change may be elucidated by this model, particularly with reference to hormonal effects on collagen and ground substance. We would also like to correlate findings related to cervical compliance with changes in electrical conductance, such as those being studied by Dr. Kriewall.

Our model for measuring cervical compliance is admittedly not yet feasible to apply to the human cervix, principally because the cervical canal in women is so much shorter in length than in the ewe. Direct measurement of compliance in the human may be technically difficult to obtain. The balloon design would have to be changed considerably. We had problems using ours in an occasional sheep with a short canal, although it was still several centimeters longer than a long human cervix. Design is, therefore, very critical.

If compliance were found to be correlated with some other measurement, such as conductance, we could then examine human cervical tissue for changes in that parameter and thereby be able to study compliance indirectly. This would have potentially important application in investigations dealing with the onset of labor or with premature labor.

REFERENCES

1. Danforth, D.N. The fibrous nature of the human cervix, and its relation to the isthmic segment in gravid and nongravid uteri. *Am. J. Obstet. Gynecol.* 53:541, 1947.
2. Danforth, D.N. The distribution and functional activity of the cervical musculature. *Am. J. Obstet. Gynecol.* 68:1261, 1954.

3. Danforth, D.N., Buckingham, J.C., and Roddick, J.W., Jr. Connective tissue changes incident to cervical effacement. *Am. J. Obstet. Gynecol.* 80:939, 1960.

4. Bryant, W.M., and Weeks, P.M. Alterations in collagen organization during dilation of the cervix uteri. *Surg. Gynecol. Obstet.* 126:27, 1968.

5. Danforth, D.N., Veis, A., Breen, M., et al. The effect of pregnancy and labor on the human cervix: Changes in collagen, glycoproteins, and glycosaminoglycans. *Am. J. Obstet. Gynecol.* 120:641, 1974.

6. Kleissl, H.P., Van Der Rest, M., Naftolin, F., et al. Collagen changes in the human uterine cervix at parturition. *Am. J. Obstet. Gynecol.* 130:748, 1978.

7. Golichowski, A.M. Changes in cervical connective tissue glycosaminoglycan composition during pregnancy. Society for Gynecologic Investigation, 25th Annual Meeting, Atlanta, Georgia, March 15-18, 1978. *Abstract No. 125,* p. 75.

8. Frieden, E.H., and Hisaw, F.L. The biochemistry of relaxin. *Recent Prog. Horm. Res.* 8:333, 1953.

9. O'Byrne, E.M., Sawyer, W.K., Butler, M.C., and Steinetz, B.G. Serum immunoreactive relaxin and softening of the uterine cervix in pregnant hamsters. *Endocrinology* 99:1333, 1976.

10. Sherwood, O.D., Chang, C.C., Bevier, G.W., and Dziuk, P.J. Radioimmunoassay of plasma relaxin levels throughout pregnancy and at parturition in the pig. *Endocrinology* 97:834, 1975.

11. Sherwood, O.D., Chang, C.C., Bevier, G.W., et al. Relaxin concentrations in pig plasma following the administration of prostaglandin $F_{2\alpha}$ during late pregnancy. *Endocrinology* 98:875, 1976.

12. Sherwood, O.D., Wilson, M.E., Edgerton, L.A., and Chang, C.C. Serum relaxin concentrations in pigs with parturition delayed by progesterone administration. *Endocrinology* 102:471, 1977.

13. Pinto, R.M., Rabow, W., and Votta, R.A. Uterine cervix ripening in term pregnancy due to the action of estradiol-17β. *Am. J. Obstet. Gynecol.* 92:319, 1965.

14. Liggins, G.C., Fairclough, R.J., Grieves, S.A., et al. The mechanism of initiation of parturition in the ewe. *Recent Prog. Horm. Res.* 29:111, 1973.

15. Hindson, J.C., Schofield, B.M., and Turner, C.B. The effect of a single dose of stilbestrol on cervical dilatation in pregnant sheep. *Res. Vet. Sci.* 8:353, 1967.

16. Najak, Z., Hillier, K., and Karim, S.M.M. The action of prostaglandins on the human isolate non-pregnant cervix. *J. Obstet. Gynaecol. Br. Comm.* 77:701, 1970.

17. Dingfelder, J.R., Brenner, W.E., Hendricks, C.H., and Staurovsky, L.G. Reduction of cervical resistance by prostaglandin suppositories prior to dilatation for induced abortion. *Am. J. Obstet. Gynecol.* 122:25, 1975.

18. Weiss, R.R., Tejani, N., Israeli, I., et al. Priming of the uterine cervix with oral prostaglandin E_2 in the term multigravida. *Obstet. Gynecol.* 46:181, 1975.

19. Conrad, J.T., and Ueland, K. Reduction of the stretch modulus of human cervical tissue by prostaglandin E_2. *Am. J. Obstet. Gynecol.* 126:218, 1976.

20. Mackenzie, I.Z. The effect of oxytocics on the human cervix during midtrimester pregnancy. *Br. J. Obstet. Gynaecol.* 83:780, 1976.

21. Fitzpatrick, R.J. Dilatation of the uterine cervix. *Symposium on the Fetus and Birth.* London: Ciba Foundation, 1976, pp. 31-47.

22. Calder, A.A., Embrey, M.P., and Tait, T. Ripening of the cervix with extra-amniotic prostaglandin E_2 in viscous gel before induction of labour. *Br. J. Obstet. Gynaecol.* 84:264, 1977.

5 Applied Physiology: The Challenge

Emanuel A. Friedman

The current era of intensive investigation of human gravid uterine physiology is now just three decades old. It has been an extremely productive period. Literally thousands of studies have been done. Their published results have slowly elucidated how the pregnant uterus works. Today, as a consequence of this frenetic activity, we have available to us a wealth of valuable information detailing the full panoply of myometrial function. It ranges from the biochemistry of subcellular contractile elements, the interrelationships of these elements to yield alteration in myofibrillar structure, and the modifications in milieu and energy sources to enhance or cycle this reaction, at one extreme, to data on a myriad of endocrine, neuronal, bioelectrical, biophysical, and grosser mechanical phenomena, at the other.

Indeed, we are privileged to know a great deal about the uterus as an organ of vital interest to us as scientists and as humanists. Yet, it withholds many of its secrets from us. In this regard, it is still very attractive as a subject for further study—and somewhat mysterious, most particularly to the clinical or applied researcher. There is a distinct separation and contrast between the rather thoroughly explored basic research domain and the almost entirely unchartered seas of clinical experience. It has been difficult at best to apply the concepts derived from the laboratory specimen of myometrial strips or even the isolated intact organ to the integrated uterus functioning within the patient, and specifically within the patient in labor.

Our global understanding of the labor processes is painfully limited. No matter how much we have learned about the nuances of uterine contraction over the last 30 years, we are still unable to distinguish the contractility pattern of, say, true labor from false, or of abnormal labor from normal. Perhaps even more illustrative of our limited grasp is our inability to distinguish the uterine contractions of labor from those the uterus experiences episodically (usually unperceived) throughout pregnancy. We accept as an obvious truth that neither adequate cervical dilatation nor effective fetal descent—both aspects sine qua non of the process of labor—can occur normally without the impetus of uterine forces. However, there is very poor correlation between the magnitude of those forces and the effect they have on the evolution of dilatation and descent. This applies regardless of how the forces are measured.

In fact, the dissociation between the expended energy and the work that energy accomplishes is sometimes paradoxical, often unexpected and disconcerting, and always without rational explanation. Quite widely disparate contraction patterns appear to be able to effect almost the same results in terms of dilatation and descent in different women. Moreover, rapid progress may be seen with relatively poor contractions, while dilatory progress may occur even in the presence of especially good contractions, everything else being equal.

Further, during the course of a given labor, abrupt acceleration of dilatation generally takes place unassociated with any appreciable change in the contractions as observed objectively or perceived subjectively. This probably reflects intrinsic changes occurring within the cervix, perhaps related to the integrity of the ground substance and/or collagen (see Chapter 4) and mirrored in sudden diminution in cervical resistance to centrifugal stretch. Although as yet unproven in the human, it is conceivable that the cervix, thus altered, can readily yield to a contractile force that it had effectively resisted earlier.

But there are other documented examples of the dissociation between uterine contractions and the dilatation process that are incapable of being argued away (as yet), even by conjecture. For example, the reduced contractile forces associated with conduction anesthesia appear entirely capable of maintaining the foregoing rate of progression in dilatation if the anesthesia is properly administered. The adverse effect of regional block peridural anesthesia on the descent process reflects its obtunding the perineal reflex and thereby its ability to inhibit the effectiveness of bearing down, a matter unrelated to our discussion here. Another example: oxytocin administered to a patient with a specific type of protraction disorder in which dilatation is abnormally slow will enhance the contractions but will not influence those improved contractions to speed the dilatation process.

Empirical observations of the dilatation and descent functions that I have been involved with for 25 years—particularly as they relate to elapsed time in labor—have served the clinician by characterizing normal progression. They offer a means for diagnosing clinical abnormalities as they arise in a simple and objective manner. They have identified obvious etiologic factors. They have fostered evaluation of management programs. They have even been useful in assessing the effects of various pharmacologic agents on the course of labor. Regrettably, however, they have provided no insight whatever into pathogenetic mechanisms. Nor have they helped us to comprehend the relation between contraction force and resultant progress. Thus, we must continue to search, in the hope of soon uncovering sufficient information to bridge this critical gap in our understanding.

6 Intrauterine Pressure Waveform Characteristics: Potential Use for Monitoring Uterine Contractility in Labor

Joseph Seitchik
Robert H. Hayashi

It is established clinical knowledge that the intrauterine resting pressure, the amplitude, and the repetition frequency of the intrauterine pressure wave are valuable measures for the study of clinical physiology and pharmacology and for the clinical management of labor. The question we have been asking is, Are there other parameters of the intrauterine pressure which could provide useful information? Before this question could be pursued, two preliminary tasks were necessary: we needed (1) to provide a precise definition of a contraction (Figure 28), and (2) to select waveform parameters for analysis.[1]

Our work is "off-line" and retrospective. All data from patients in the same clinical state were grouped into single sets. Three groups of patients were studied: (1) patients in spontaneous labor, (2) those with hypocontractility treated with oxytocin, and (3) those patients with oxytocin and prostaglandin inductions of labor.[1-3]

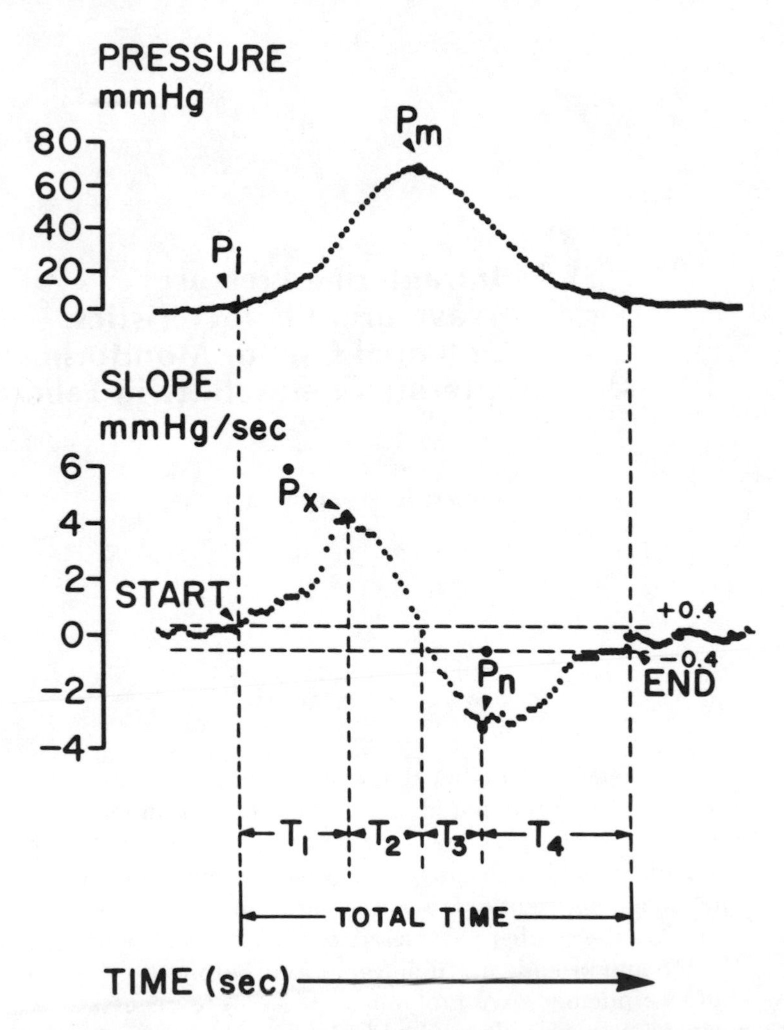

Figure 28. Digitized intrauterine pressure waveform (top) and first derivative (bottom). An arbitrary threshold is established at ±0.4 mm Hg/sec. A contraction starts on the first second after the rate exceeds the threshold, and the intrauterine pressure value at the moment equals P_i. Rate must persist above the threshold for 5 sec. The maximum of the first derivative ($\dot{P}_x$) defines the end of interval T_1. The maximum pressure (P_m) is defined as the intrauterine pressure at the first negative value of the first derivative, which also denotes the end of interval T_2. Similarly, the minimal value of the first derivative ($\dot{P}_n$) terminates the interval T_3. Contraction is completed on the first second after the first derivative exceeds the low threshold value, providing the first derivative remains within the threshold for 8 sec or exceeds the upper threshold.

The average values for amplitude, resting pressure, and duration of contractions obtained from patients in active spontaneous labor were similar to those obtained by others from oscillograph records.[4,5] This assured us that our techniques for filtering, analyzing, and storing these data were not distorting the results.

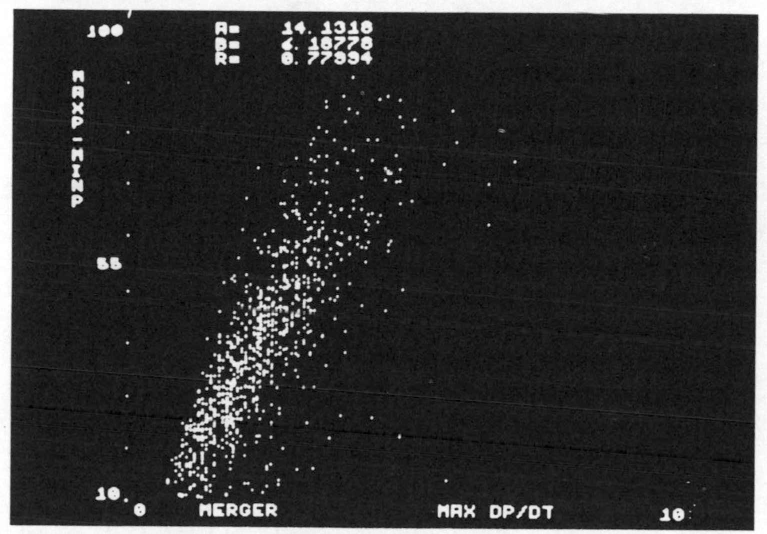

Figure 29. The amplitude of each contraction (MAXP-MINP) is plotted on the Y-axis (mm Hg), and the maximum rate of rise (MAX DP/DT) on the X-axis (mm Hg/sec) for more than 900 contractions from 23 patients in active-phase first stage of spontaneous labor.

The relationship of amplitude (P_m-P_i) to the maximum rate of rise of the pressure ($\dot{P}_x$) was linear for individual patients (Figure 29), and for each clinical group as a whole. Examination of the ratio of amplitude to the maximum rate of rise, $(P_m - P_i)/\dot{P}_x$, over the whole range of amplitudes, suggested that the relationship was curvilinear reaching an asymptote (Figure 30). Oxytocin altered the ratio of amplitude to the maximum rate of rise because oxytocin increased the maximum rate of rise disproportionately. $PGF_{2\alpha}$ produced the same results as spontaneous labor. Thus, it appears that, in this respect, oxytocin produces contractions different from those of spontaneous or $PGF_{2\alpha}$-induced labor.

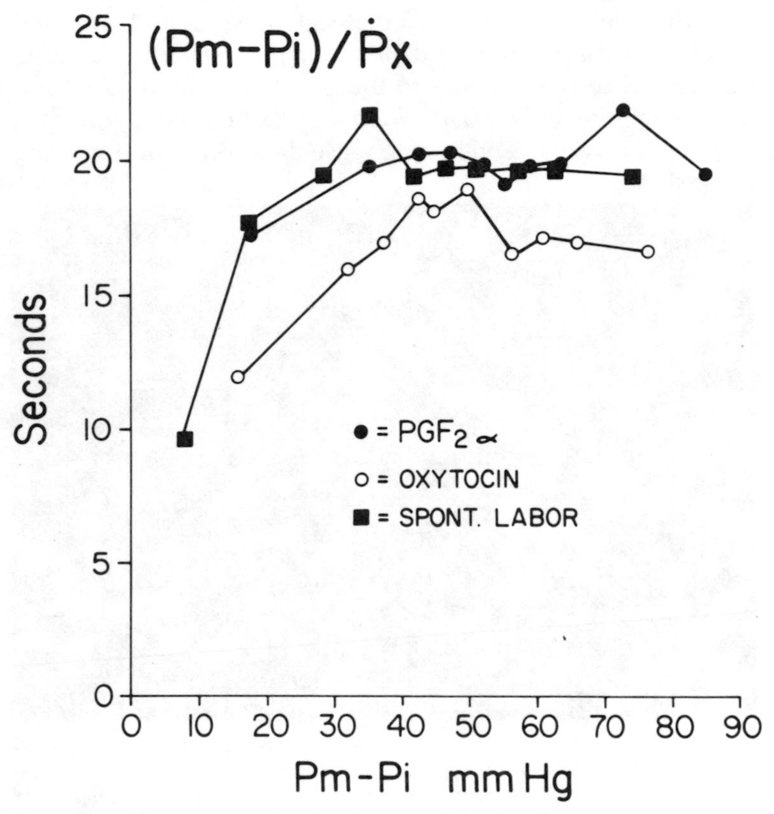

Figure 30. The average values for the ratio of amplitudes to maximum rate of rise (Y-axis) are plotted against the average values for decile subsets of the amplitude (X-axis) for patients in active-phase labor. Spontaneous, oxytocin-induced, and $PGF_{2\alpha}$-induced labors are shown separately.

Examination of the duration of the contraction and its segments indicated that the relationship between the duration of contraction and the amplitude was curvilinear. The midportion of the contraction (T_2, T_3) appeared invariate with amplitude, but the start-up and termination times increased in curvilinear fashion with increased amplitude (Figure 31). Oxytocin appeared to shorten T_1, but it had no disproportional effect on T_4 in respect to amplitude (Figure 32).

In summary, oxytocin-stimulated contractions appeared different from those of spontaneous labor in three ways: $\dot{P}_x$ was

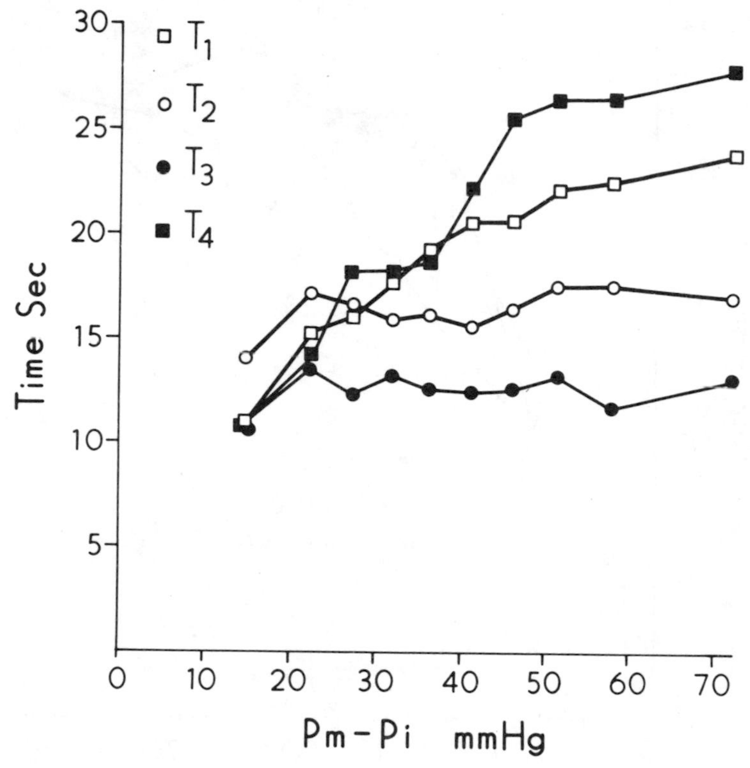

Figure 31. The averages for the time segments defined in Figure 28 (Y-axis) are plotted against the average values for decile subsets of the amplitude (X-axis).

disproportionately large in respect to amplitude; thus, the ratio of $(P_m\text{-}P_i)/\dot{P}_x$ was disproportionately low. The difference in the ratios was most evident at amplitudes greater than 50 mm Hg. T_1 appeared shorter with oxytocin.

If these additional parameters could be applied in selecting the minimal effect of a dose of oxytocin, or in recognizing changing sensitivity to the drug, or in anticipating overdoses, they would be most useful. However, before these observations can be used in clinical management, it is necessary to demonstrate that these results, observed thus far in data derived from groups of patients, can also be found in individual patients. The analysis presented is anecdotal and retrospective. The methods used are identical with those

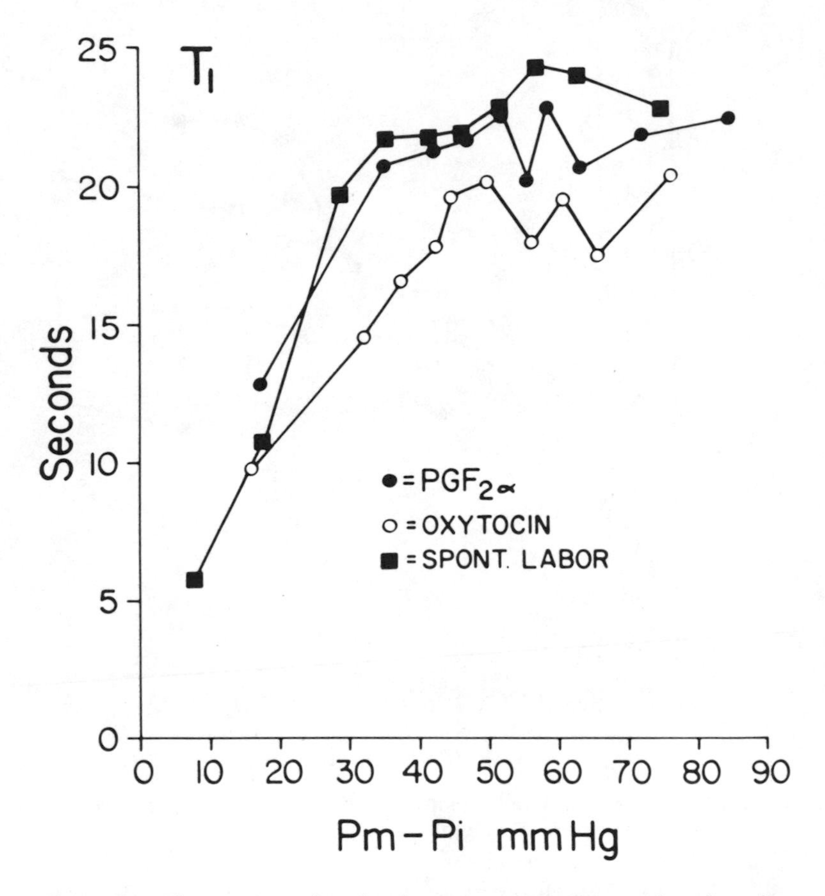

Figure 32. The average values for the start-up time, T_1, are plotted on the Y-axis against the average values for decile subsets of the amplitude for patients in active-phase of spontaneous, oxytocin-induced, and $PGF_{2\alpha}$-induced labors, respectively.

reported previously, except that digital filtering (24 db at 0.07 Hz) and a four-point moving average are used to smooth the data; a threshold value of ±0.2 mm Hg/sec is used to identify the start and end of a contraction. Clinical data and the several parameters of the intrauterine pressure waveform are presented for three illustrative cases in graphic form (Figures 33 through 38).

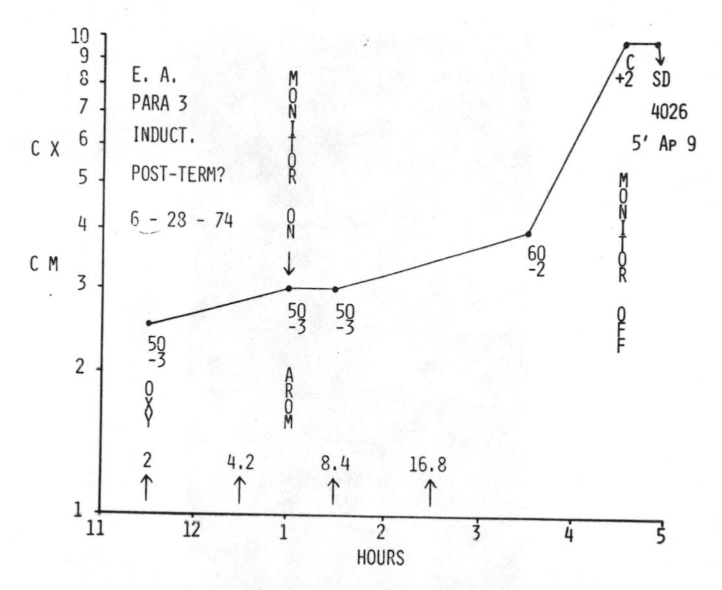

Figure 33. Clinical course of Case No. 500. The patient is a para 3, possibly postterm. When she presented, her cervix was 2 to 3 cm dilated, 50% effaced, and the fetal station was − 3. Induction was initiated with oxytocin given at 2 mU/min and increased to 4.2, 8.4, and 16.8 mU/min at the times shown. Internal monitoring was initiated at 3 cm cervical dilatation after artificial rupture of the amniotic sac (AROM), and was terminated at complete dilatation (C). Patient successfully delivered (SD) a 4026 gm infant, Apgar score 9 at 5 min.

COMMENT

The dose-response curve of the human uterus to oxytocin is curvilinear with a tendency to reach an asymptote.[6] When the dose is increased in some regular progression in respect to time, the results are similar to those obtained in dose-response curves.[7] As a result of the curvilinearity, the maximal dose of oxytocin used is usually at least two increments larger than the dose necessary to achieve effective contractility. In some patients, excessive contractility results. The therapeutic situation is complicated further in successful labors because the myometrium changes its sensitivity to oxytocin as labor progresses. This is evidenced by the fact that in at least one-third

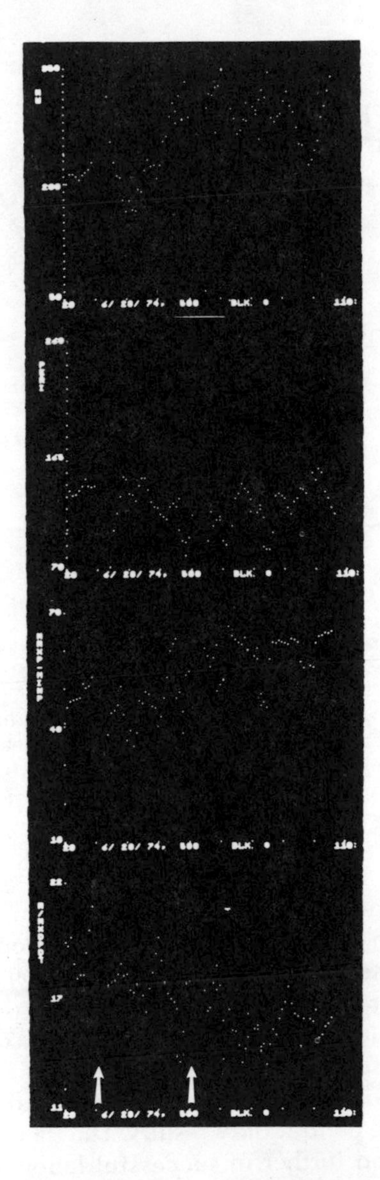

Figure 34. Case No. 500. The data for Montevideo Units (MU), period (PERI), amplitude (MAXP-MINP), and the ratio of amplitude to the maximum rate of pressure rise (A/XDPDT) are plotted (Y-axis) against elapsed time (X-axis) from the initiation of monitoring. Each time interval between the dots on the X-axis equals 21 1/3 min. The arrow on the left denotes the approximate time of in-

crease in oxytocin to 8.4 mU/min and the arrow on the right, to 16.8 mU/min. There are brief periods just prior to the first arrow and just after the second when there are no data. This is the result of patient manipulation required for patient hygiene or care which distorts signals beyond the capacity of the filtering system used. The following observations are made: The amplitudes of contraction present two different steady state periods. The first approximate one-third of the record contains contractions that are generally in the range of 40 to 50 mm Hg. This is followed by a transition to another steady state where most of the amplitudes range from 55 to 65 mm Hg. Period does not appear to be affected by the oxytocin at 8.4 and 16.8 mU/min, with most values ranging from 110 to 150 sec. The Montevideo Unit values follow the amplitude. In contrast, the values for the ratios of amplitude to maximum rate rise of the pressure follow a consistent pattern. Most values are in the range of 17.5 to 19.5 sec on 4.2 mU/min, 16.5 to 18.0 sec on 8.4 mU/min, and 14.0 to 16.5 sec on 16.8 mU/min. The overall trend is a progressive decline as the oxytocin dose is increased.

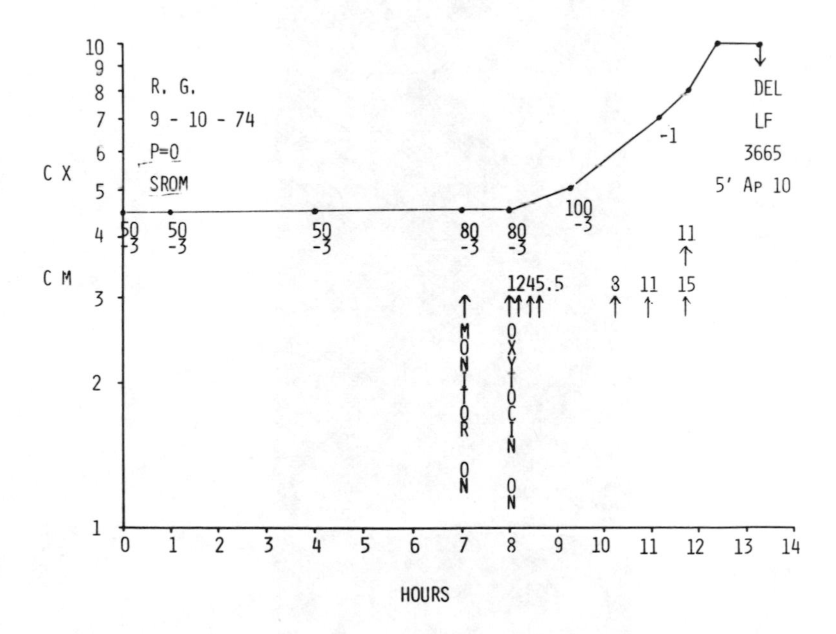

Figure 35. Clinical course of the labor in Case No. 585. The patient is a nullipara with spontaneous rupture of the membranes. Induction with oxytocin was initiated with the cervix 4 to 5 cm dilated, 80% effaced, and vertex presentation at station − 3. Internal monitoring was begun one hour prior to oxytocin and continued the full dilatation. Patient experienced spontaneous delivery of a 3665 gm infant. Oxytocin was initiated at 1 mU/min and rapidly increased in incremental fashion to 5.5 mU/min and later to 8, 11, and 15 mU/min as shown.

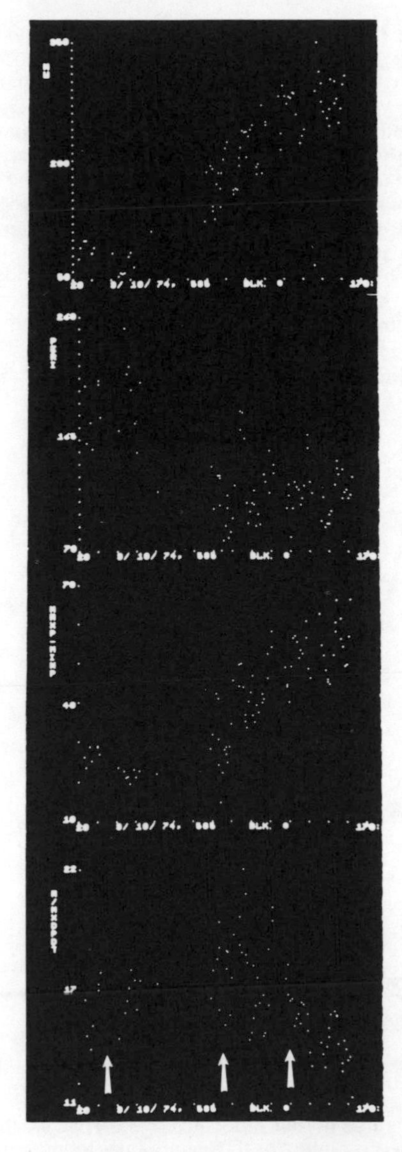

Figure 36. Case No. 585. The data are displayed as in Figure 34. The arrow to the left denotes the initiation of oxytocin therapy; the middle arrow identifies the increase to 8 mU/min, and the arrow to the right, 15 mU/min. There is a period of approximately 40 min just prior to the middle arrow when there are no data. The following observations are made: Prior to the administration of oxy-

tocin, most values for A/XDPDT were 15 to 17 sec; amplitude, 20 to 30 mm Hg; period, 150 to 210 sec; 70 to 100 Montevideo Units (MU). During the first 42 minutes of oxytocin therapy, there is no significant change in any of these values. After the period of absent data but *prior* to the increase in dose to 8 mU/min, the majority of values for A/XDPDT exceeds 17 sec, although the majority of amplitude values are equal to or less than 30 mm Hg. Period values have fallen to 80 to 130 sec, and Montevideo Units range from 100 to 200. Prior to the dose of 15 mU/min, amplitude ranges from 40 to 60 mm Hg; period, approximately 110 to 130 sec; Montevideo Units, 220 to 270. A/XDPDT values range from 16 to 22 sec; 15 mU/min produces only slight further increase in amplitude to 45 to 65 mm Hg and 250 to 300 MU, little change in period, but decrease in A/XDPDT to 12 to 16 sec.

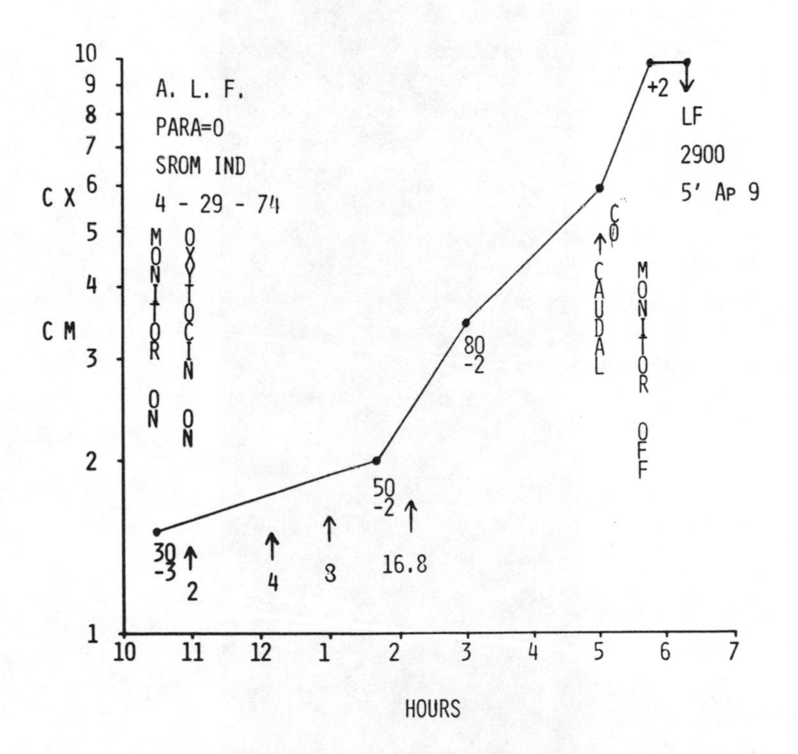

Figure 37. Labor course of Case No. 340. The patient was a nullipara induced for spontaneous rupture of the membranes. At the time the monitoring was begun, the cervix was 1 to 2 cm dilated and 30% effaced, with the fetal vertex at station − 3. Oxytocin was administered in doses of 2, 4, 8, and 16.8 mU/min, as shown. Caudal anesthesia was administered at 6 cm of cervical dilatation. Monitoring was stopped at full dilatation. The patient was delivered of a 2900 gm fetus by low forceps (LF).

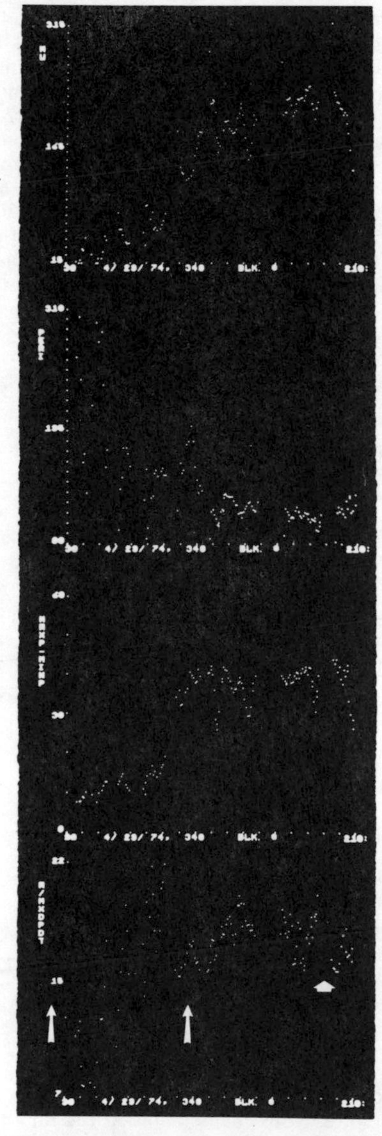

Figure 38. Case No. 340. The data are displayed as in Figure 34. The large arrow to the left indicates the initiation of oxytocin; the arrow of similar size to the right indicates the time the largest dose, 16.8 mU/min, was started; the short arrow to the right indicates the start of caudal anesthesia. The values for A/XDPDT rise to levels found in satisfactory contractility, 16 to 22 sec in the interval prior to achieving a steady state response in either amplitude or

of induced labors oxytocin may be discontinued at 5 cm of cervical dilatation without affecting the labor progress. If it is not discontinued, the dose necessary to maintain labor is usually significantly less than that required to initiate it.[8]

Most large obstetrical services experience cesarean section rates of 10% to 15% these days. More than one-half the primary operative procedures are performed for "failure to progress." The vast majority of these cesarean sections have been preceded by a trial of oxytocin therapy. In this clinical state, the sine qua non for the evaluation of first stage labor progress, cervical dilatation, does not occur at a satisfactory rate; and the criteria for selection of the maximum oxytocin dose are the intrauterine pressure parameters, amplitude, and repetition frequency, not cervical dilatation. The recommended [9] end points are three or more contractions per ten minutes, 50 mm Hg or more amplitude, and 200 Montevideo Units. These exceed the average values for 85% of normal spontaneous labors.[4,5]

Our retrospective analysis of 20 oxytocin-induced labors or oxytocin-treated hypocontractile labors demonstrated only a single instance in which the ratio of amplitude to the maximum rate of rise did not reach its maximum value or a steady state prior to the other parameters reaching their maxima or steady states. In the examples of induced labors we have presented, it is clear that the ratio of amplitude to the rate of pressure rise identifies the myometrial response to oxytocin earlier than amplitude or Montevideo Units. This ratio is a more sensitive dose-response indicator than period, which changes little with increasing doses once a steady state is achieved. These observations suggest that the ratio of amplitude to the rate of the intrauterine pressure may be a useful measure for monitoring oxytocin therapy, but proof of its utility awaits prospective studies.

Montevideo Units. The shortening of the time between contractions to 180 sec or less accompanies the change in values for the ratio, A/XDPDT. Caudal anesthesia had no effect on any of the intrauterine pressure parameters.

DISCUSSION

Dr. Melvin Barclay: Could you tell us why you used a four-contraction moving window for your calculations rather than the time interval in which the contractions occurred? We have used a somewhat different algorithm and have been especially troubled by the problem of variability. We have been able to reduce it somewhat by establishing different time frames according to the degree of variability we see.

Dr. Seitchik: We have no great brief for this approach. It was intended to provide a variant of the Montevideo Unit for computer application. We could have looked at ten blocks of 128 seconds to determine how much uterine activity was present. Our technique allowed us to pursue a means for computing our data readily and simplistically. It has no special advantage other than convenience. We accept the inevitability of variability, but we are most concerned with examining different aspects of the pressure curve of the contraction, rather than its frequency in a given interval.

Dr. Work: How can one define a uterine contraction objectively? This is a commonly asked question among residents in training.

Dr. Seitchik: Clinically, a contraction is one that produces a detectable change in intrauterine pressure. As a "circular" definition, this is less than perfectly satisfactory. For our purposes, a contraction was defined when it met the minimum criteria of a given rate of change in pressure over a specified time interval, namely, an increase of at least 0.2 mm Hg per second. This definition, while admittedly arbitrary, has proven quite useful to us, although it is not absolutely reliable at all times.

Parenthetically, I do not believe the waveform pattern necessarily reflects whether or not the patient will be able to deliver vaginally. Using this method, we examined a series of patients who were being given oxytocin for failure to progress in labor and who were ultimately subjected to cesarean section. There was no consistent pattern in the parameters we studied either before and after oxytocin to help predict the final outcome. Hypocontractility was not uncommonly associated with obstructed labor. The waveform of the contractions tended to be unrelated to the goals of the contraction, specifically, cervical dilatation and effacement.

Dr. Noah: Could you postulate the physiologic significance of your observations? How do the various parameters relate to what we see clinically?

Dr. Seitchik: Most of the investigation done so far on the physiologic correlation of muscle function to mechanical behavior of an organ has dealt with the heart. The force developed as related to the rate at which that force develops turns out to be very constant. For the uterus, I doubt the existence of a pacemaker or conduction system. Among the billion muscle cells in the uterus, those that are going to engage in a given contraction will all start to do so within about three seconds of each other. What we see in our approach basically reflects what all these cells are doing together. When prostaglandin is given, the contractions still follow the same behavior pattern as spontaneous contractions.

However, when oxytocin is administered the result is different. T_1 is shortened; the rate at which the contraction pressure builds is disproportionately increased; the rest of the waveform is unchanged. Thus, the termination components are the same with oxytocin-induced contractions as for those occurring spontaneously or after prostaglandin-$F_{2\alpha}$.

If we accept the concepts that Dr. Carsten has described, perhaps we see here differences in calcium release and return on the biochemical level. If this is correct, oxytocin affects calcium transport differently, and the oxytocin-induced contraction is the result of a substantive pharmacologic difference, perhaps yielding an importantly different contractile state. This is not to suggest the result is bad merely because it is different. I hope I will not be misinterpreted in this regard.

Dr. Friedman: There is a commonly held belief among clinicians that oxytocin regularizes uterine contractions. We often see the contractile pattern, as obtained by external tokodynamometry or by internal strain gauge, develop a monotonous uniformity, each contraction form looking precisely like the previous one. This contrasts with spontaneous uterine contractions, which appear quite heterogeneous and at times almost disordered in pattern. I could not fully appreciate this kind of difference in your records. Could you clarify that?

Dr. Seitchik: I do believe it was present. We see some approximation of the steady state with oxytocin. This is particularly the case when we examine the standard deviations for given intervals; they diminish as the variability falls. There is regularization in association with oxytocin, but not as much as one would expect or like to see.

We have studied the rhythmicity of contractions with techniques comparable to those used for analyzing arrhythmias in cardiac intensive care units. A computer is employed to assess beats in terms of the interval between them. The plot of points for a patient not in active labor tends to be fairly randomly distributed. By contrast, active labor yields a more regularized field, whereas oxytocin stimulation provides a display of relatively fixed intervals.

REFERENCES

1. Seitchik, J., and Chatkoff, M.L. Intrauterine pressure waveform characteristics of spontaneous first stage labor. *J. Appl. Physiol.* 38:443, 1975.

2. Seitchik, J., and Chatkoff, M.L. Intrauterine pressure waveform characteristics in hypocontractile labor before and after oxytocin administration. *Am. J. Obstet. Gynecol.* 123:426, 1975.

3. Seitchik, J., Chatkoff, M.L., and Hayashi, R.H. Intrauterine pressure waveform characteristics of spontaneous and oxytocin or prostaglandin-$F_{2\alpha}$ induced active labor. *Am. J. Obstet. Gynecol.* 127:223, 1977.

4. Shulman, J., and Romney, S. Variability of uterine contractions in normal human parturition. *Obstet. Gynecol.* 36:215, 1970.

5. Anderson, G., and Schooley, G. Comparison of uterine contractions in spontaneous or oxytocin or $PGF_{2\alpha}$-induced labors. *Obstet. Gynecol.* 45:284, 1975.

6. Poseiro, J.J., and Noriega-Guerra, L. Dose-response relationships in uterine effects of oxytocin infusions. In R. Caldeyro-Barcia and H. Heller (Eds.). *Oxytocin.* New York: Pergamon Press, 1961.

7. Steer, P.J., Little, D.J., Lewis, N.L., et al. Uterine activity in induced labour. *Br. J. Obstet. Gynaecol.* 82:433, 1975.

8. Beazley, J.M., Banovic, I., and Feld, M.S. Maintenance of labour. *Br. Med. J.* 2:248, 1975.

9. Miller, F. Uterine activity, labor management and perinatal outcome. *Sem. Perinatology* 2:181, 1978.

7 Some Effects of the Forces of Labor on Cervical Dilatation and the Fetal Skull*

Timothy J. Kriewall

Parturition is a dynamic process involving the interaction of certain structures that behave as a system. Energy is put into the system by the contractions to make the system change its state. Since energy can neither be created nor destroyed, much can be said about a system by observing how the input energy is redistributed throughout the system during its work cycle.

Traditionally, this is the manner of engineering analysis; whether it is an automobile, a refrigerator, or a living system, a machine can be analyzed by observing how the energy flow is

*The effects of labor on cervical dilatation were developed in clinical collaboration with Bruce A. Work, Jr., MD. The effects of labor on fetal skull molding were developed in collaboration with Gregg K. McPherson, PhD. This work was made possible with the financial support of The University of Michigan's Division of Research and Development Administration, a Horace Rackham School of Graduate Studies Faculty Development Award, The University of Michigan's Medical School Fund for Computing, and The University of Michigan's Biomedical Research Support Grant.

conveyed from the input to the output. Our research emphasis is to learn more about parturition by observing certain input/output relationships with instrumentation and analytical techniques in more than an empirical manner. Theoretically developed and time-proven laws of mechanical structure analysis, thermodynamics, and electric field theory, coupled with certain assumptions about the behavior of the structure, are applied in both data gathering and analysis. It is the intent of this paper to show that this engineering analysis approach is both applicable and insightful in the study of parturition.

Since the prime mover of labor is the contraction, it can be classified as the system input. Two recipients of the input energy are the cervix and the fetal head. The change in their states can be classified as the system outputs. The input/output relationships between these fetomaternal system parameters will be the subject of this chapter.

THE FORCES OF LABOR ON CERVICAL DILATATION

The dynamics of cervical dilatation dictate that it must be measured continuously. With each contraction the cervix dilates, but after the contraction subsides the cervix returns to near its before-contraction state (Figure 39). Monitoring pressure and dilatation continuously provides more information about the dynamics and progress of parturition than intermittent checks of the dilatation state via the pelvic examination.

We have just recently developed a second-generation instrument to monitor dilatation continuously. A very small magnetic field source and a magnetic field sensor are attached to diametrically opposite edges of the cervix. The field source is comprised of two small electromagnets oriented 90° with respect to each other. They are excited with electrical currents that are also 90° out of phase. This has the effect of producing a field at the sensor which is minimally affected by the angular orientation between the source and sensor. Thus, the field strength at the sensor is only a function of the distance which separates the source and sensor. The electronics of the instrument convert the field strength to separation and display the

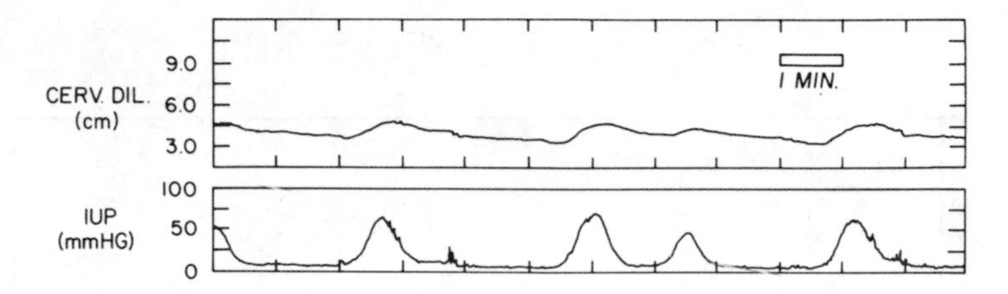

Figure 39. With each contraction, the cervix dilates but returns close to its precontraction state after the contraction subsides. The degree of dilatation with each contraction depends on the condition of the cervix, the strength of the contraction, and the stage of labor.

distance in centimeters on a panel meter. In addition, the pressure and dilatation are displayed side-by-side on a strip chart recorder and are recorded as voltages on an FM tape recorder. These latter signals are used in the computer processing of the waveforms after labor is complete.[1]

As most people who use medical instrumentation appreciate, the most difficult problem with its use is interfacing the instrument to the patient. The current technique to attach the transducers to the cervix is by means of small suction cups. We are not completely satisfied with this method in that small vacuum lines must run to the suction cups. In addition to suction cups, we have used helical scalp electrode needles and various spring clip arrangements, each having its own set of problems. Our present work includes developing a more satisfactory and unobtrusive means of attachment that permits easy application.

With the equipment in place, we can observe certain characteristics that may have an effect upon the future outcome of labor. In particular, the temporal relationship between the pressure and dilatation waveforms may indicate cervical dystocia or cephalopelvic disproportion, and there exists a synergistic relationship between pressure and dilatation that can be used to calculate uterine efficiency.

The peak of dilatation generally does not occur at the same time as the peak of the pressure. Rather, the cervix continues to dilate for a period of time even as the pressure is subsiding. The delay, or time lag between waveform peaks, varies typically between four and ten seconds (Figure 40).

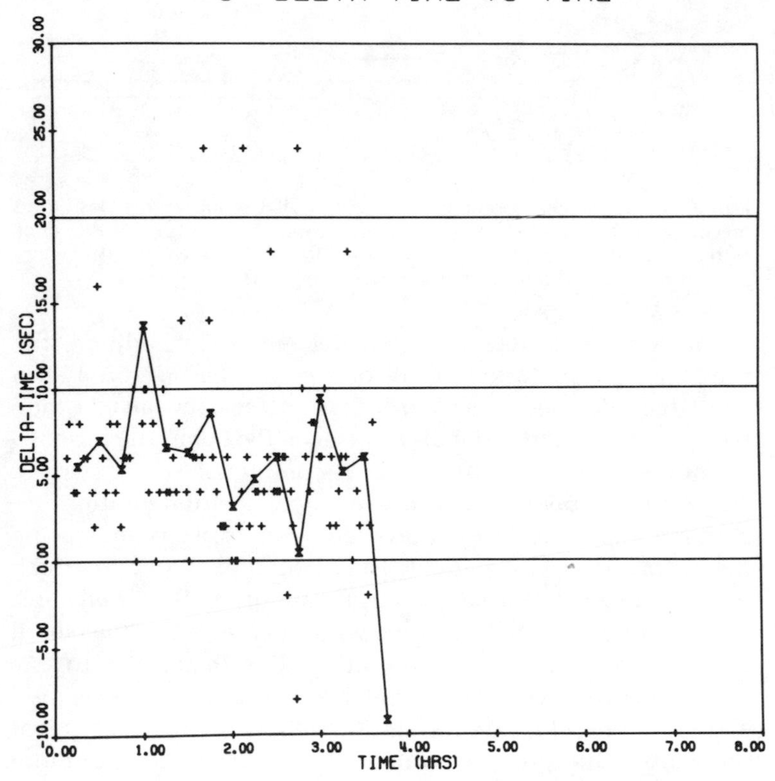

Figure 40. The peak of the dilatation waveform typically follows the peak of the contraction waveform by four to ten seconds as demonstrated by this scatter diagram of delays for a particular labor. This diagram was generated by processing the tape recorded pressure and dilatation waveforms on a computer after the labor was complete.

This time lag could be an indicator of the likelihood that a given labor will result in a vaginal delivery. As the contraction develops, the overall length of the uterus is shortened, the cervix retracts and the fetal presenting part pushes against the cervix and soft tissues of the maternal pelvis. In the case of cervical dystocia or cephalopelvic disproportion, an extended time lag may not appear. A balance of forces must exist between the downward forces pushing on the fetus and the upward viscoelastic forces of the cervix and pelvic tissues pushing back of the fetus. When no cephalopelvic disproportion is present, the cervix will continue to dilate and the fetus will descend into the pelvis until a balance of forces is met.

After this point, the elastic forces of the stretched cervix and compressed maternal soft tissues will have the effect of pushing the fetus back into the uterus. With cervical dystocia or cephalopelvic disproportion, the upward forces will be invoked sooner due to the increased resistance opposing descent and/or retraction. Therefore, a balance of forces will be reached sooner in the pressure cycle. The cervix will stop dilating sooner with the resulting peak of dilatation occurring nearer the peak of the contraction, perhaps even exhibiting a phase lead. In summary, we will be observing the temporal relationship between the pressure and dilatation waveforms as a potential prognosticator of the delivery method.

Another relationship exists between the pressure and dilatation waveforms that enables us to assess the uterine energy being expended to dilate the cervix. Since energy can neither be created nor destroyed, all energy put into the system is either stored within the system or transferred out of the system in the form of heat and/or work. The energy dissipated during the contraction is in several forms: (1) heat transferred from the myometrium to the maternal blood (Q), (2) heat buildup in the cervix due to nonelastic tissue resistance (W_R), (3) potential energy in the stretched elastic fibers of the cervix (W_E), and (4) work performed by the uterus.

The work performed is of two types: the work required for brachystasis (the shortening and thickening of the uterine wall) and the work required to expel the internal contents of the uterus (W_{dV}). With present-day techniques, the work of brachystasis is incalculable, but the work of expelling the uterine contents can be estimated. Mathematically, it is defined as the integral of the internal pressure times the incremental change in volume, or:

$$W_{dV} = \int_{V_2}^{V_1} P \, dV$$

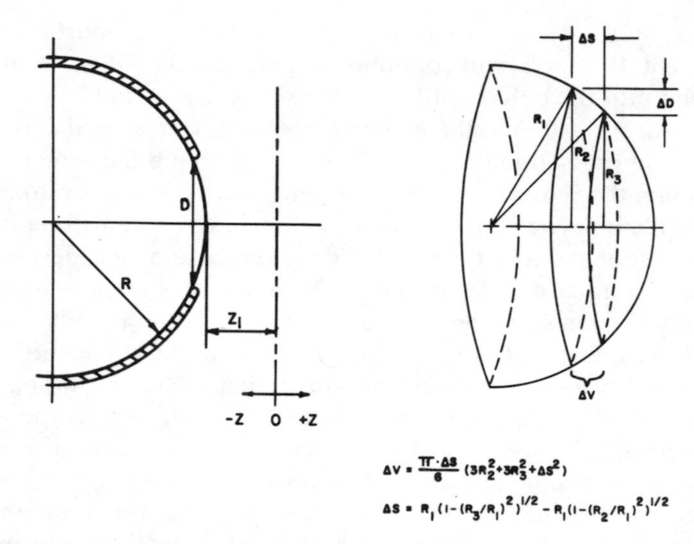

Figure 41. An approximation of the presenting part as a hemisphere permits the calculation of uterine volume change directly from changes in cervical dilatation, assuming the cervix is in contact with the presenting part. Other geometries (eg, an ellipse) can also be used to simulate the presenting part.

If the fetal presenting part is approximated by a given geometry (eg, a hemisphere or a hemiellipse), the change in uterine volume, dV, is a function of the change in dilatation. Referring to Figure 41, we can derive the following expression:

$$dV \cong \Delta V = \pi \cdot \Delta S(3R_2^2 + 3R_3^2 + \Delta S^2)/6,$$

where $\Delta S = R_1[1 - (R_3/R_1)^2]^{1/2} - R_1[1 - (R_2/R_1)^2]^{1/2}$

and $R_1 = 5$ cm

A similar expression is derivable if an ellipse is used to approximate the presenting part. Solving these equations numerically on a computer permits assessment of the energy expended contraction by contraction in dilating the cervix (Figure 42). By observing the expended energy over the course of labor, we can see that normal labor is a rather homeostatic process, as demonstrated in Figure 43—that is, the energy expended by contractions late in labor is approximately the same

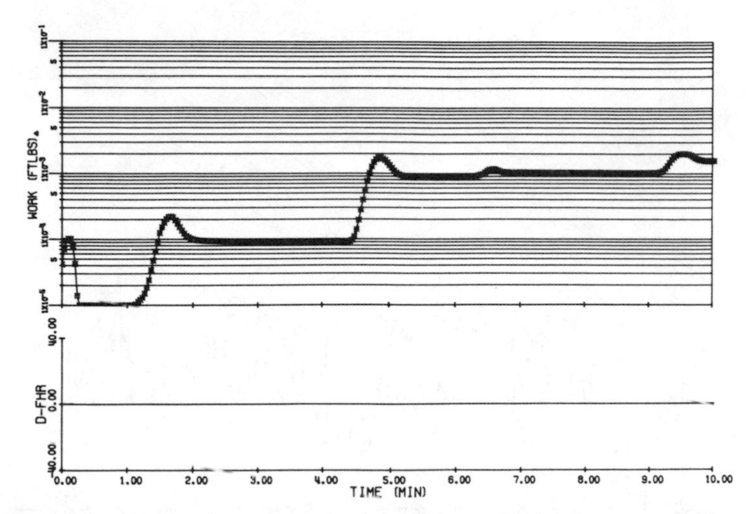

Figure 42. With each contraction, energy is expended by the uterus to dilate the cervix. The energy that is expended in dilating the elastic portions of the cervix is returned to the fetomaternal system after the contraction subsides, leaving a net amount of work expended to dissipative forces.

as that in early labor, even though the change in dilatation with each contraction continually diminishes during the active phase of labor (Figure 44).[2] On the other hand, when a laboring mother begins to reach the limit of her energy reserves, we would expect to see a diminution of the energy expended with each contraction.

Utilizing these concepts, we can describe efficiency of labor in thermodynamic terms. Efficiency is defined as the work sought divided by the energy that it costs. The work sought is W_{dV}; the energy that it costs is $Q + W_R + W_E + W_{dV}$ (ignoring the work of brachystasis). The heat transferred, Q, is theoretically derivable but requires us to measure the temperature difference between the myometrium and maternal blood as well as the uterine blood flow. Therefore, Q is impractical to calculate. Another way of defining efficiency might be to remove Q from the efficiency equation and use the following expression for efficiency instead:

$$\text{Efficiency} = \frac{W_{dV}}{W_{dV} + W_E + W_R}$$

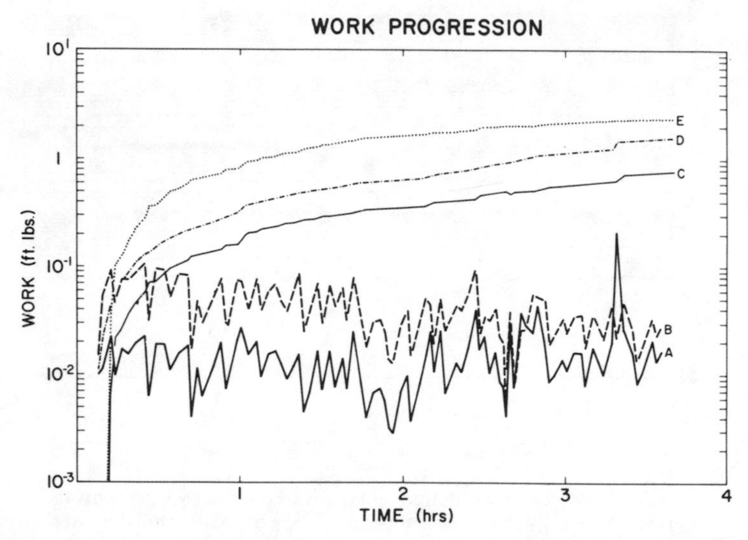

Figure 43. Curve A plots the net work expended contraction by contraction using a hemisphere of diameter 10 cm to simulate the presenting part (ie, the difference between plateau values in Figure 42). Curve B is the net work expended when an ellipse having a major diameter of 14 cm and a minor diameter of 10 cm is used to simulate the presenting part. Curve C is the cumulative sum of A. Curve D is the cumulative sum of the gross energy expended in dilating the cervix, corresponding to the difference from a plateau value to the subsequent peak value in Figure 42. Curve E is the cumulative sum of B.

Referring to Figure 43, we find this term is closely approximated by the abscissa of C divided by the abscissa of D for the same point on the ordinate. From Figure 43, the uterine efficiencies for this patient at one, two, and three hours could be calculated to be 0.53, 0.51, and 0.55, respectively.

THE FORCES OF LABOR ON THE FETAL SKULL

Another structure to which energy is transmitted by the forces of labor is the fetal skull. In magnitude, the amount of energy is probably insignificant compared to that mentioned above, but from the viewpoint of fetal welfare, the energy being transmitted to the fetal head can be crucially important in cases of cephalopelvic disproportion, low-slope active

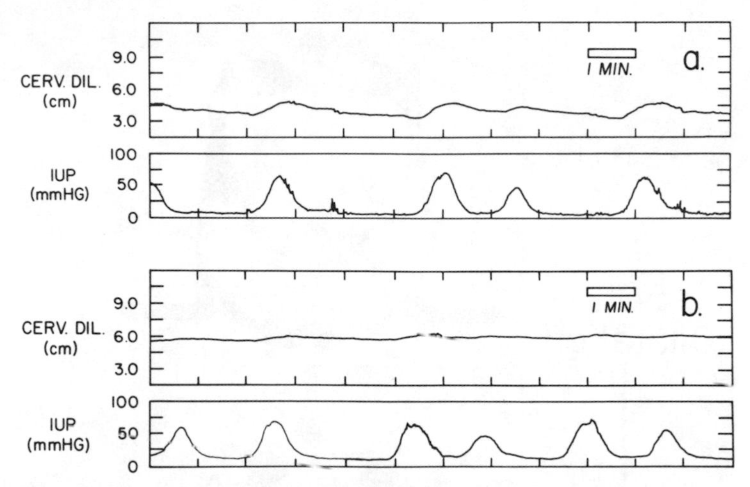

Figure 44. Although the change in dilatation diminishes with each contraction as labor progresses (from a to b), the energy expended remains fairly constant (see Figure 43).

phase labor, secondary arrest labor, and premature labor. In order to characterize the input/output relationship between the uterine contractions and the fetal head, we have begun a project to quantify the energy needed to mold a fetal head.

By simply observing a neonate's molded head after delivery, we cannot say much about how the head took on that shape. In a radiographic study, Borell and Fernstrom[3] documented that molding, like dilatation, is a dynamic process. Figure 45 summarizes how the head assumes its final shape after delivery. First, during pregnancy, Braxton Hicks contractions flatten the head.[4] With the onset of labor, the head is forced against the cervix, bending the parietal bones at the vertex and decreasing the biparietal diameter. At complete dilatation, the circumferential forces are maximum in a plane cutting through the parietal eminences. At this point, the biparietal diameter is a minimum. With complete dilatation and descent, the cervix is in the suboccipitofrontal plane. The frontal and occipital bones are flexed in, locking at their respective sutures with the parietal bones. The resultant effect is a lifting of the occipital bones. At this point, the head assumes an elongated shape compared to its antepartum state.

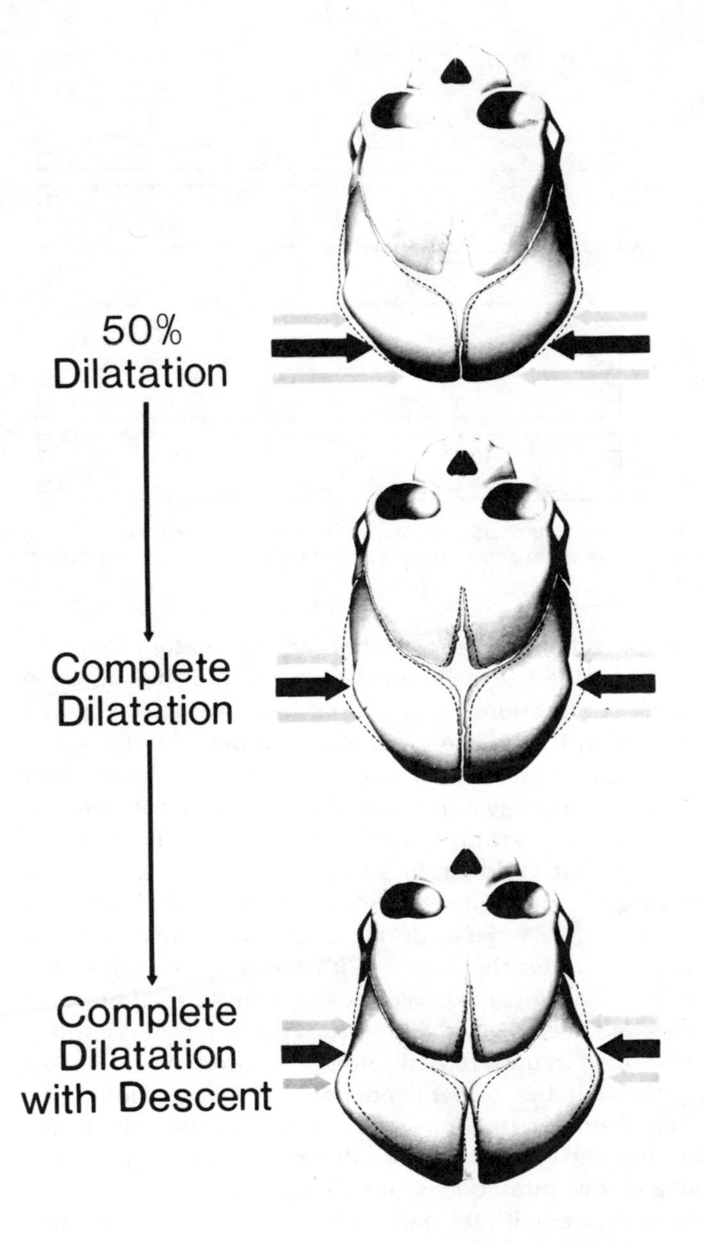

Figure 45. Skull molding is a dynamic process that involves numerous movements of the bony plates as they pass through the birth canal. Dotted lines

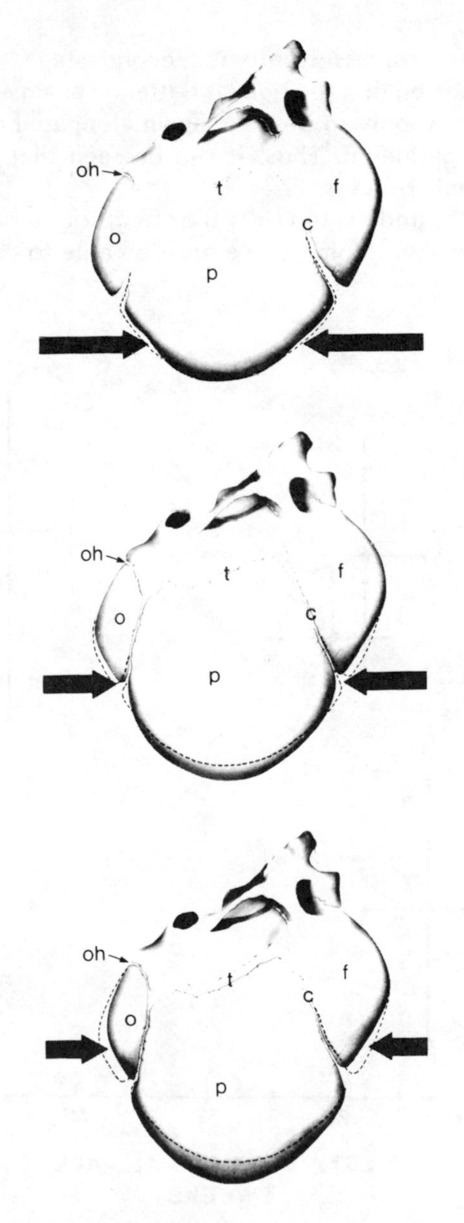

represent unmolded head. *f:* frontal bone; *p:* parietal bone; *o:* occipital bone; *c:* coronal suture; *t:* temporal suture; *oh:* occipital hinge.

As labor progresses into its second stage, Borell and Fernstrom showed that the head is flattened again as it reaches the pelvic floor, only to be once again elongated as it passes through the perineum. Thus, it can be seen that molding is itself a dynamic process.

In order to understand fully the effects of uterine contractions on fetal skull molding, we must be able to characterize

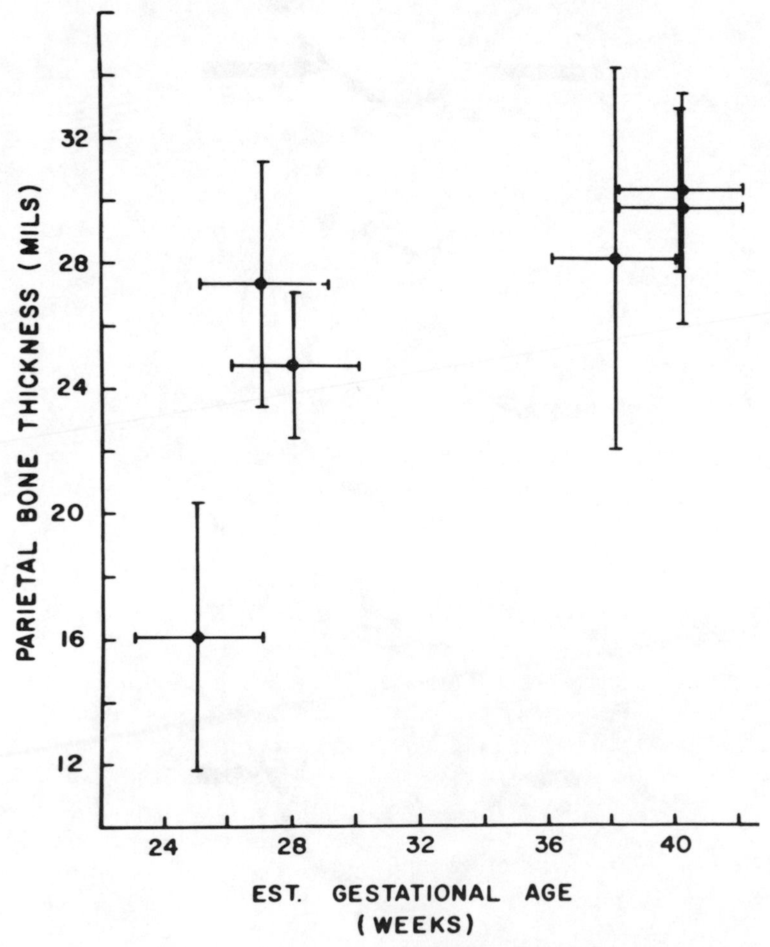

Figure 46. The thickness of the parietal bone increases during the gestational period; the thickest portions are at the parietal eminences and the thinnest at the outer margins.

the geometry of the head, know the pressure magnitudes that are being exerted on the head, and know the material properties of the underlying, load-bearing structures (viz, the skull bone and dura mater). With this information, a mathematical model can be formulated to simulate the effects of the labor forces. A good model can also be used to diagnose the degree of skull molding during labor.

The geometry of the skull is fairly quantifiable. Through the work of Lindgren[5] and Schwarcz et al.,[6] the intrapartum pressures have already been measured. Therefore, we began our project by quantifying the material properties of the head's stiffest structure, the cranial bone.

Our goal was to assess the bone's modulus of elasticity, an index of the material stiffness. Small specimens (1.0 × 0.08 in) were cut from calvaria of neonates that had died of causes that would not affect the bone's material properties. Experimental conditions were controlled to keep the specimens representative of living tissue.

Two immediate findings of our study were that fetal skull bone thickness varies directly with gestational age (Figure 46) and that fetal skull bone exhibits a pronounced fiber orientation (Figure 47). In order to characterize the mechanical properties of the bone adequately, we felt we had to take these two

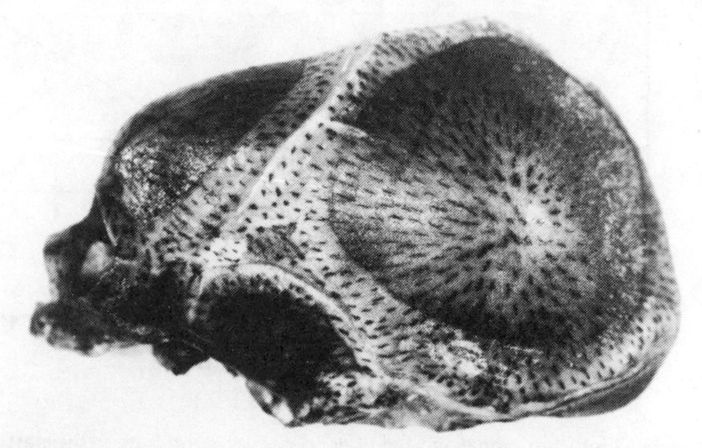

Figure 47. The skull bones of the fetus have a pronounced fiber orientation, as demonstrated by split lines of ink droplets that follow the grain structure.

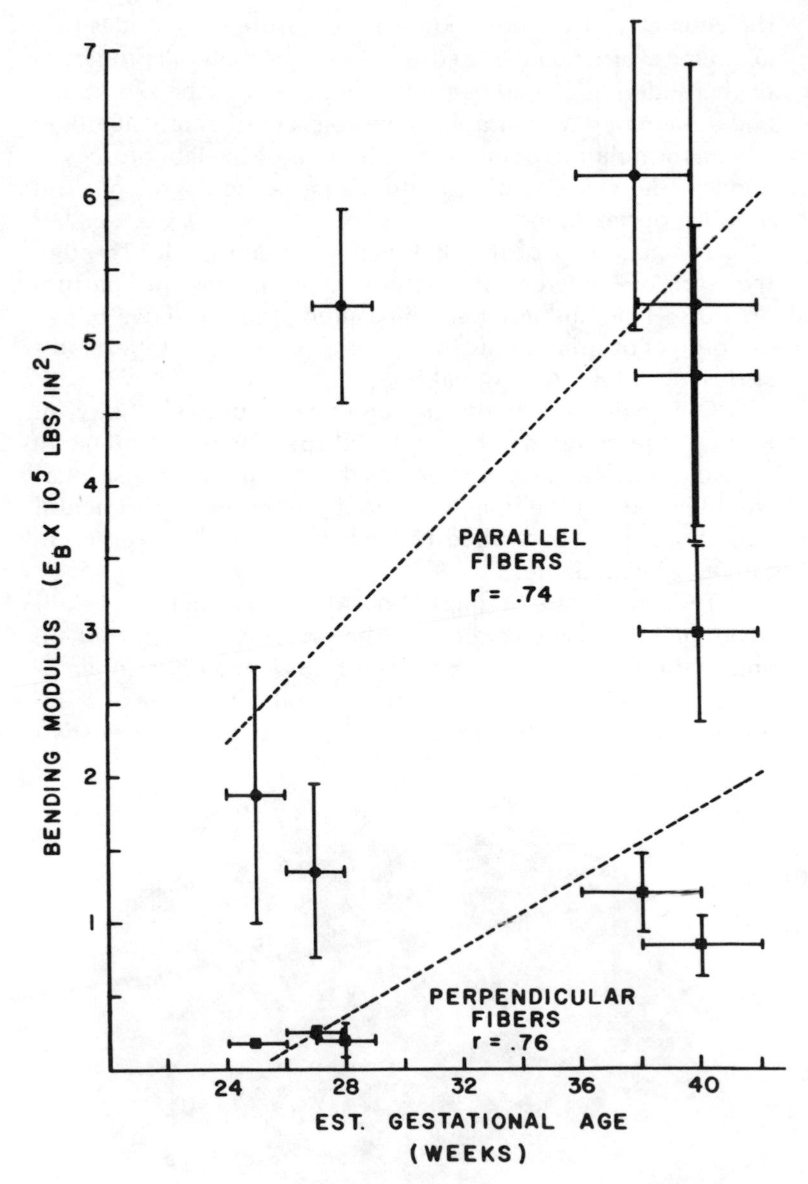

Figure 48. Both gestational age and fiber orientation contribute to the elastic modulus in bending. The vertical bars represent ±1 SD of the mean value of the measured moduli of samples from the same calvarium; the horizontal bars represent the range of estimated gestational age.

independent variables into account. Cross-sectional dimensions were accurately measured on all test specimens and normalized out in calculations for the bending modulus of elasticity. In addition, the specimens were cut from the calvaria so that their long dimensions were, for the most part, either parallel or perpendicular to the fiber orientation.

Mechanical testing on the specimens showed a marked dependence on the fiber orientation (Figure 48). The stiffness (ie, bending modulus) was significantly greater ($p < 0.001$) in those specimens cut parallel to the fiber orientation. In addition, the bending modulus was significantly greater ($p < 0.001$) for term infants as compared to preterm infants. The average bending modulus for term infants was 1.38×10^5 lbf/in^2 and for term infants, 0.21×10^5 lbf/in^2. This fact may account for the increased risk of brain damage due to birth trauma that the premature infant faces.

A mathematical model of the fetal head was formulated using the above statistics and a technique called finite-element analysis, which is employed by engineers to characterize structures. A structure, for example, a bridge (Figure 49), can be broken into a number of straight-line elements. Each element can be given its own set of material properties, usually those tested in a laboratory. The interaction of all the elements can then be observed as the entire structure is subjected to any kind of prescribed load. This is typically performed on a computer because most structures of significance can be modelled only by a large set of finite elements.

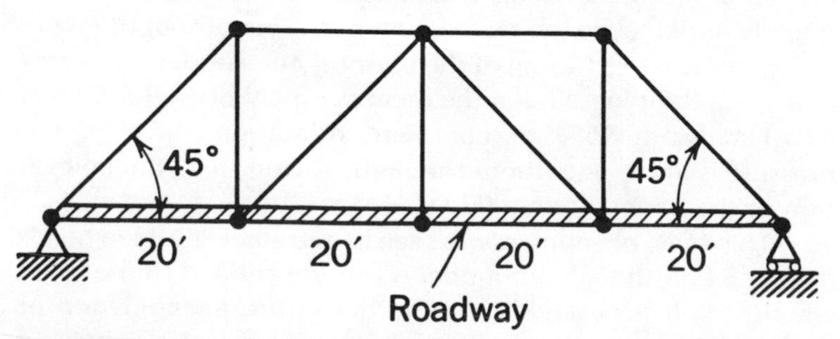

Figure 49. Finite-element analysis requires a structure to be broken into straight-line elements, a straight-forward task for this bridge structure.

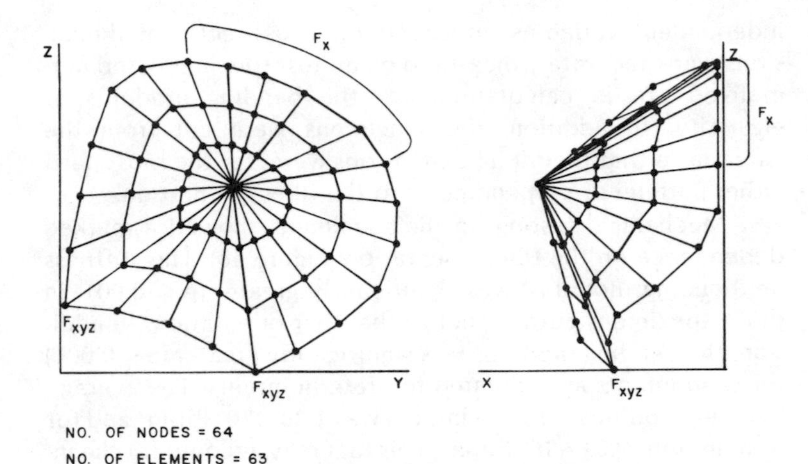

NO. OF NODES = 64
NO. OF ELEMENTS = 63

Figure 50. A finite-element model must be more complex for structures with irregular shapes, as for a parietal bone.

Using this same analysis technique, we modelled a parietal bone by a set of finite elements, as shown in Figure 50. Applying the loads found clinically by Lindgren and by Schwarcz, the model predicts the following deformations. During the intrapartum period, a uniform hydrostatic pressure of approximately 50 mm Hg is exerted on the head. The resultant deformation is a flattening of the head, giving rise to a diminution of the mentovertical diameter (Figure 51). At approximately 50% of complete dilatation, the pressures at the vertex of the head were assumed nil; but at the internal os, the pressures are higher than the intrauterine pressure and rise linearly until they reach a maximum at the equator of the skull. This gives rise to a flexing of the parietal bone about the vertex and a resultant increase in the mentovertical diameter (Figure 52). Finally, at 95% of complete dilatation, most of the pressure is at the equator of the skull, causing a distinct elevation of the parietal bones (Figure 53).

This same phenomenon is seen in extremely molded heads (Figure 54). Although our model is not yet refined to the point where it will accurately describe the entire phenomenon of skull molding, we can see that it does show promise of being a very useful tool. If the head can be characterized by a model

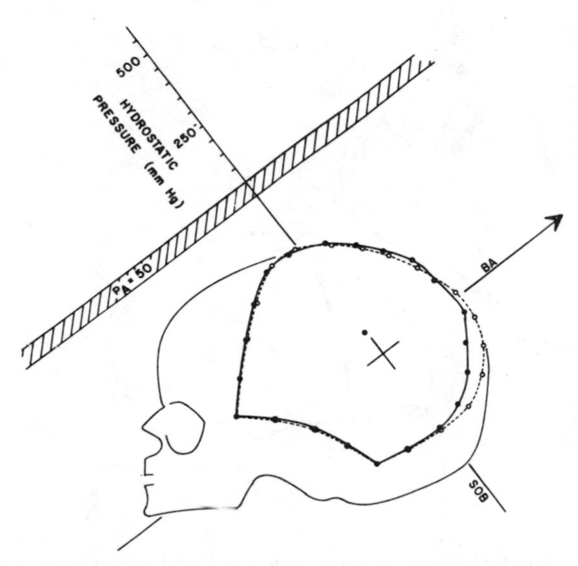

Figure 51. The predicted deformation of a term parietal bone under constant hydrostatic pressure. The deformations are shown twice actual size for clarity. SOB: suboccipitobregmatic plane; BA: axis of birth canal.

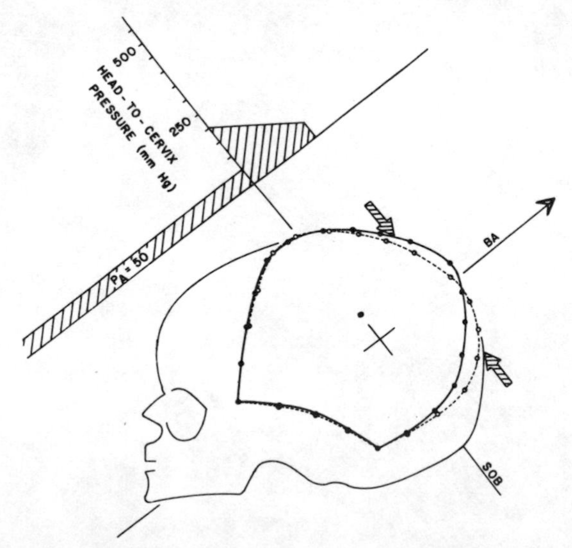

Figure 52. The predicted deformation changes for 50% cervical dilatation, mainly accounted for by an increased flexing at the vertex.

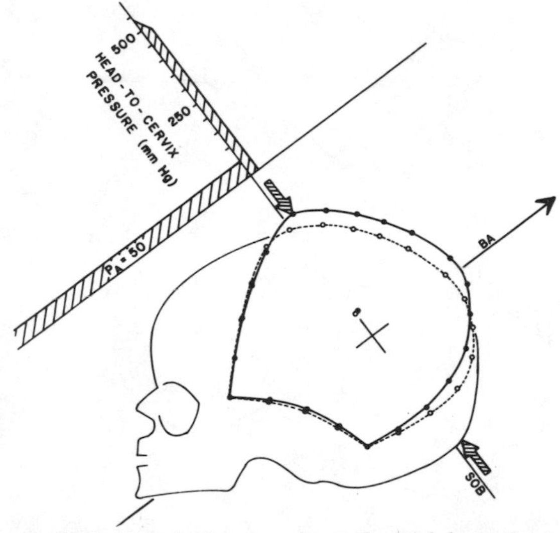

Figure 53. At 95% cervical dilatation, the predicted deformation results from an elevated parietal bone.

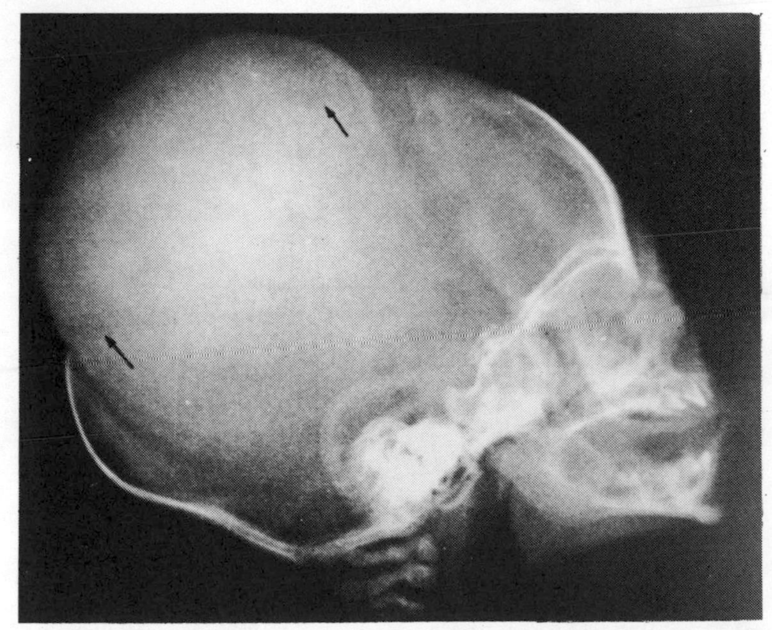

Figure 54. Displacement of the parietal bones, as predicted by the finite-element model, is often seen in severely molded heads. Lateral x-ray view of a newborn infant.

with life-like material properties, then monitoring of intrapartum pressures will indicate the degree of intrauterine deformations. Thus, the degree of skull molding can perhaps one day be monitored continuously during labor to ensure that brain damage will not be a consequence of birth trauma.

CONCLUSION

Our goal is to quantitate physiologic parameters of parturition that are indicative of labor's progress and labor's effect on the fetus. In particular, the temporal relationship between intrauterine pressure and cervical dilatation may be indicative of the future course of labor. The calculation of uterine work can be used to estimate uterine efficiency. Application of engineering analysis can show what effects the forces of labor have on the fetal skull. For example, our data indicate that the premature infant is at greater risk of neurologic trauma than its term counterpart, due to a less developed cranium, allowing greater calvarium strains (ie, molding). Finally, by applying the material properties found in our testing, we have developed a mathematical model to approximate the behavior of the bony plates of the head as they are subjected to pelvic pressures. The course of our future research will be to define this model better so that the degree of molding might be diagnosed during the intrapartum period.

DISCUSSION

Dr. Stys: In your investigation of bending modulus of the cranial bone, have you quantitated the forces necessary to produce the degree of molding seen to occur in your model?

Dr. Kriewall: The forces we found were very comparable to those measured by Lindgren and by

Schwarcz et al. We assumed the pressure distribution they reported and observed the degree of change the distributions produced in the model head. The mechanical properties we observed in actual fetal skulls yielded dimensional changes quite similar to those shown by Borell and Fernstrom in their radiographs, thus verifying their independent observations. The pressures on the skull, however, are not the same as the hydrostatic pressure within the uterus. They increase at the cervical os up to high levels at the major diameters of the fetal head. Lindgren showed them to increase to as high as 200 mm Hg at the equator of the head; although Schwarcz disagreed with the absolute magnitude, he too found that they increased.

Dr. Friedman: Can this important information be translated into meaningful clinically applicable relationships? For example, at what point does external surface contouring of the fetal skull become a critical manifestation of what may be happening inside the head, specifically with regard to the integrity of the falx cerebri or the tentorium cerebelli. At what point is the stretch modulus exceeded to the point of lacerating a critical structure within the fetal cranium to produce irreversible damage? I assume it is too early in your investigative program to provide the answers, but I am encouraged to believe your approach may ultimately yield such data.

Dr. Kriewall: We have undertaken this program one step at a time and, thus far, only the first parts have been completed. We have gathered data on the stiff structures and are moving toward examining the soft tissue quantitatively. We will seek what is called the "yield point," which refers to the conditions of strain at which the tentorium will give way. We expect to look at tissue specimens in just the same way we looked at the calvarium to determine mechanical properties. Except for the national space program and some highway safety research, little work has been done on soft tissues other than aorta and dura mater. Nobody else seems to be especially concerned with what is happening to the fetus. We intend to correct this oversight.

Dr. Friedman: You may have made some basic assumptions that could be called into question. Apposition of the fetal head appears to be an essential element in your model for functional dilatation of the cervix. If so, it can be challenged on the basis of several recognized clinical circumstances in which dilatation occurs in response to uterine contractions without such a fetal relationship. These include cases with insurmountable cephalopelvic disproportion, those with the fetus presenting in transverse lie, and the rare missed labor in an abdominal pregnancy. Although there is no fetal presenting part apposing the cervix (and even nothing at all in the uterus in one of these conditions), cervical dilatation can and does take place.

Dr. Kriewall: In each of these special instances, it is apparent that fetal head apposition is not a relevant factor in the development of cervical dilatation. We can postulate that the uterine volume can change by a mechanism of myometrial retraction or brachystasis. This implies that one component of energy is here related to both elastic and resistive aspects of the process. Other components include that energy dissipated in the form of heat or in changing the uterine configuration, just as they might include the energy required to change the configuration of the fetal skull. Although these last items are assumed to be negligible by comparison with the uterine volume component, we are now in a position to begin to measure some of them, particularly the energy expended in cranial molding, because we have material parameters we can use for calculation. If it proves to be negligible, it will help throw some light on these issues.

Dr. Barclay: Your early observations showed intrauterine pressure rising before the cervix begins to change. This suggests that there is an isometric phase to uterine contraction which may allow some very interesting things to go on in terms of modelling. This has not been reported before.

Dr. Kriewall: I do not know why it has not been recognized in earlier studies. Could it be explained by differences in the sensitivity of instrumentation? In the clinical event, the volume of the system must remain constant for a finite period of time, specifically during the latent phase of labor, during false labor, during Braxton Hicks contractions, and perhaps even throughout the course of pregnancy. Clearly, contractions must be isometric at times.

Dr. Work: There is now obvious wide interest in gentler and safer childbirth. Could you comment on how intact membranes might influence the output of your model?

Dr. Kriewall: We have given this some thought, but we have not yet studied the problem experimentally. At first, we thought amniotomy might augment the process, but it is clear that an intact forebag will not help much in effecting cervical dilatation if the fetal skull is in direct contact immediately behind it. On the other hand, if the membranes constitute a cushion of fluid between the head and the pelvis, they may act like a balloon or shock absorber, perhaps acting to alter the mechanical factors involved in both cervical dilatation and cranial molding. It is going to require further objective study before we have any definitive answers.

Dr. Work: Do you have any ideas as to how clinicians will ultimately be able to monitor the degree of fetal head molding that is occurring during the course of a given labor? It is apparent that your investigations must focus our attention in this area, bringing a very complex laboratory model into a real-life clinical setting.

Dr. Kriewall: Obviously, what is important to the clinician is his ability to assess when molding may be reaching some excessive value. He must be able to make measurements of the fetal skull during labor. Ultrasound scanning by current techniques are inadequate because the maternal bony pelvis is an impediment to good imaging. Cineradiography is unacceptable because it will continually expose the fetus to x-radiation. Thus, we cannot serially observe the dynamic changes in the fetal head.

The best we have right now, in our present state of technology, is intrapelvic pressure measurements, especially the pressure determinations between the fetal head and the cervix at various levels. If we can characterize the mathematical relationships—as we have tried to do with our fairly crude model—and ascertain the mechanical properties of the head, this information may enable us to project what dimensional changes can be expected for given pressures. This may have special relevance in a situation characterized by disproportion between the head and the pelvis, bearing directly on an important clinical application. Temporal factors undoubtedly have special relevance here as well. Pressure can be expected perhaps to build up much more quickly in association with cephalopelvic disproportion than in its absence.

Dr. Friedman: It would seem possible that some of the energy dissipated in the living model is utilized in the course of a contraction for dislocating the uterus within the abdomen. We recognize, for example, that the fundal portion of the uterus rises forward in the supine laboring patient, provided her abdominal wall is sufficiently relaxed to permit it to do so. If the abdominal wall integrity prevents the uterus from anteflexing during a contraction, perhaps this energy is dissipated in heat. May we assume you are thus far unable to measure this aspect of energy loss?

Dr. Kriewall: Yes, our calculations of efficiency are only reasonable approximations. We are ignoring a few identifiable, but unmeasurable, factors which we cannot as yet handle on the assumption that some information is better than none. Your point is well taken, however, because it reminds us to be cautious in how we analyze our data and, more importantly, how we interpret the results of such analyses.

REFERENCES

1. Kriewall, T.J., and Work, B.A., Jr. Measuring cervical dilatation in human parturition using the Hall effect. *Med. Instrumentation* 11:26, 1977.

2. Kriewall, T.J. Uterine work in parturition. *J. Appl. Physiol.* 41:316, 1976.

3. Borell, U., and Fernstrom, I. Die Umformung des Kindlichen Köpfes Wahrend Normaler Entbindungen in Regelrechter Hinterhauptslag. *Geburt. Frauenh.* 18:1156, 1958.

4. Kriewall, T.J., Stys, S.J., and McPherson, G.K. Neonatal head shape after delivery: An index of molding. *J. Perinatal Med.* 5:260, 1977.

5. Lindgren, L. The causes of foetal head moulding in labour. *Acta Obstet. Gynecol. Scand.* 39:46, 1962.

6. Schwarcz, R.L., Strada-Saenz, G., Althabe, O., et al. Compression received by the head of the human fetus during labor. In *Physical Trauma as an Etiological Agent in Mental Retardation.* Washington, D.C.: U.S. Department of Health, Education and Welfare, 1970.

8 Directions for Future Activities

Dr. Friedman: Our overall review has been exceedingly edifying. Dr. Carsten began by providing us with a great amount of information to clarify how myometrial cells function. Dr. Stys followed and gave us new insights into intrinsic cervical changes associated with advancing pregnancy. Dr. Clewell did likewise with reference to the dynamics of uterine circulation. We have been privileged to hear Dr. Seitchik's valuable commentary on the significance of variables dealing with intrauterine pressure waveforms; we are hopeful that he and his coworkers will continue to evolve important relationships along these lines that will be applicable to clinical problems. Finally, Dr. Kriewall has concluded with work on mathematical models based on intrapelvic pressure, cervical dilatation, and cranial molding. These have offered us a particularly optimistic outlook, a brief but far-reaching glimpse at exciting future developments. The dynamics of the labor phenomenon are clearly adaptable to use of such mathematical models. They are especially attractive as research tools because they do not involve any further encroachment on or direct approach to the patient for purposes of gathering relevant data. In this era of growing sensitivity to patients' needs and rights, such considerations become increasingly critical. This sets the stage for us to consider our future directions.

Dr. Work: This portion of our deliberations has been left entirely unstructured. Our objective here is to free-associate, to indulge in speculations, and openly to query each other in order to attempt to correlate our several disciplines. In this way we hope to be able to provide direction for the future and suggest possible orientations in basic laboratory and applied clinical research endeavors.

Dr. Noah: Are there any data available in the human myometrium, Dr. Carsten, on the intrinsic prostaglandin concentrations at the cellular level? If there were, perhaps they would give us some better insights into the functional role of this agent and offer us a more understandable basis for clinical pharmacologic applications.

Dr. Carsten: We have tried to determine prostaglandin concentrations in our preparations, but I have to introduce a word of caution here. We are studying the cellular biochemistry of myometrium in the cow, not the human. We must not be deluded into making the broad leap of assuming that the findings in a species so remote from the human is directly reflective of what may be going on in the human. We recognize differences of great physiologic and biochemical significance even among primates. Nonetheless, in the cow, based on only a few observations, we can say that there are only minimal amounts of prostaglandin present in the cytoplasm and no appreciable synthesis under the conditions of our experiments.

In regard to a possible intercorrelation of our respective studies, I would like to have some clarification about oxytocin and its effect on uterine contractility. We have seen that oxytocin increases intracellular calcium concentration. Dr. Seitchik showed pressure waveform changes associated with the use of oxytocin characterized by increased rate of rise, but not by increased amplitude. If true, could this be a reflection of an inherent biochemical-physiologic relationship?

Dr. Seitchik: Specifically, for contractions of equal amplitude the rate of rise of the pressure is greater with oxytocin than without it. This applies with regard to both spontaneous and PGE_2-stimulated contractions. If that period during which the pressure is rising represents the interval of calcium release then it follows that oxytocin may be enhancing the rate of calcium release. Such an interpretation is logical.

Dr. Friedman: Could we take this observation one step further into the realm of clinical application? We appreciate that the essence of oxytocin administration is to enhance uterine contractions and simulate the contractility pattern of normal labor, thereby producing normal labor progression of cervical dilatation and fetal descent. In carefully controlled circumstances, this is feasible to accomplish. The real question, however, is whether or not the contractility pattern produced is the same as that of spontaneous contraction in terms of its effect on the fetus. It has been shown that the frequency of abnormal fetal heart rate patterns is increased in association with oxytocin administration, even in the absence of tetanic contractions. This suggests that oxytocin may have an adverse effect on the fetus or fetoplacental unit, perhaps mediated by way of diminution in uterine blood flow as a consequence of the augmentation in uterine contractility you have observed. Uterine contraction inhibits uterine blood flow normally, but usually without discernible impact on the fetus; is it possible that uterotonic stimulation by oxytocin—even without affecting the general pattern of contractility as defined by the usual gross clinical parameters of intensity, frequency, and duration—may further diminish uterine blood flow to beyond the critical point at which the manifestations of oxygen deprivation become apparent in the fetus?

Dr. Seitchik: Your point is very valid. There is no question but that we must be primarily concerned about the welfare of mother and fetus. It is imperative that we examine data in patients who experience such apparently adverse effects. We have to dissect the waveform patterns in a group of this nature to learn what specific contractility patterns they exhibit. Overdosage, subtly manifest or perhaps unrecognized, may be the underlying problem; alternatively, there may indeed be a distinctive pharmacologic action on the myometrium or even directly on the vessels of the uterus or the placental bed to affect blood flow and circulation. Clearly, this is an area that should be explored.

Dr. Clewell: Although we have been studying blood flow in labor, we recognize the sheep is not a very good model to help answer the issues raised. Labor in sheep is characterized by contractions of low intrauterine pressure, of about 15 mm Hg pressure, never rising above the animal's diastolic blood pressure. Thus, the critical aspect of the possible adverse effect of uterine pressure on uterine blood flow is probably not relevant here. As mentioned earlier, we must be very cautious about recognizing interspecies differences. Anyone who examines the effects of labor on uterine or placental blood flow in the sheep will obtain results that are uninterpretable for the human. As far as I know, however, the only effect that oxytocin has on uterine circulation is a mechanical one brought about as an indirect consequence of its action on the myometrium.

Dr. Seitchik: There is a growing feeling among clinicians—and I do not wish to imply that I agree—that we now are in the position of being able to monitor uterine contractility, labor progression, and fetal status so well by objective means (including fetal monitoring and Friedman curves of dilatation and descent), that subtle considerations such as these become irrelevant, academic and unimportant. Is it true that our current capability to monitor fetal status allows us to be cavalier?

Dr. Friedman: The pendulum appears to be swinging too far away from the extreme dubiety and skepticism of the past to almost total reliance and acceptance today on the value of fetal monitoring. Monitoring techniques in use today are exceedingly limited when used to assess when excessive intracranial mechanical damage may be occurring. We must stress that fetal heart rate monitoring is not at all capable of helping the obstetric attendant to recognize excessive fetal cranial molding or to anticipate an irreversible intracranial catastrophe. There is a finite period of time in the usual sequence of events after mechanical damage has taken place before intracranial bleeding begins that will result in further localized brain damage, ultimately to yield fetal hypoxia, which in turn will become manifest as a characteristic series of changes in fetal heart rate pattern. Fetal monitoring today is a splendid and delicate means, albeit indirect and somewhat limited, for detecting hypoxia in the fetus; however good it may be in this respect, it is poor at best as a measure of mechanical damage until long after the fact and often too late.

Dr. Stys: I do not think any physician would be comfortable caring for an adult patient when all the information available consisted of a heart rate recording and perhaps an occasional blood pH determination. We could tell if the patient were alive, but not too much more. Fetal movement assessment has recently been added as another indicator of fetal wellbeing. By analogy to the adult, this is like merely looking into the room from the doorway and pounding on the door to ascertain if the patient moves. It is not very reassuring information, yet it is all we have available as yet and is admittedly much more than was available in the past.

Dr. Work: There is no disagreement here. Much needs to be done to improve our ability to assess fetal status. However, there is general agreement that current monitoring techniques are very useful in providing assurance when the fetus is in good condition. Accepting that there are some false negatives in which fetuses with severe acidosis can present minimal fetal heart rate changes, by and large normal patterns are valuable indicators. Granted they do not guarantee fetal health, but the correlation between normal patterns and fetal wellbeing is so strong that we generally feel comfortable with them. On the other side of the coin, the relationship between fetal distress patterns and outcome is very poor. Not many babies with abnormal patterns will show manifestations of intrauterine hypoxia when they are delivered. The question we must address is whether or not we have a tool sufficiently sensitive to provide us with the information we need to determine whether or not we should intervene and, if we should intervene, when in relation to the appropriate time before irreversible hypoxic damage has occurred. We do not have the answer to this critical question as yet, and perhaps we never shall.

Dr. Friedman: I am strongly in agreement. We are confronted with a classic Arrowsmith dilemma (for the Sinclair Lewis readers among us), and it constitutes an unresolved, perhaps unresolvable, issue. The controlled, laboratory-designed experiment that would be required to provide us with the scientific verification we need to show the intrinsic value of fetal monitoring has never been done, and in our current climate can probably never be done. On ethical grounds, it would be immoral to withhold the technology or the information obtained by technical advances in use if such a practice could possibly be detrimental to the individual, but only by withholding it can we provide a parallel controlled group for purposes of critical comparisons. Today, we have accepted the value of fetal monitoring based on wide usage and experiential observations; to withhold it for scientific purposes is unthinkable.

Good fetal heart rate patterns correlate very closely with good infant outcomes, as shown by Schifrin[1] at our institution. Abnormal patterns correlate poorly with outcomes. The latter can be explained by the intervention that usually takes place under these circumstances. We tend to intervene aggressively to remove these fetuses from their hostile environment before they are damaged. It should not be surprising, therefore, that they are delivered in fairly good condition. We are not willing to allow such babies to succumb or to be damaged by prolonged exposure to hypoxia in utero. Before the significance of abnormal patterns was fully appreciated, intrauterine fetal death and severe damage did occur under like conditions while we stood by helplessly. But those isolated cases serve as mere testimonials, and cannot be considered to constitute irrefutable scientific evidence. Currently, such scientific documentation, while obviously needed, is probably no longer obtainable.

Dr. Stys: Along these lines, one unanswered question that demands resolution is the time sequence of hypoxic damage that may be associated with fetal heart rate abnormalities. We need to know how long it is acceptable to allow a fetus who exhibits a specific pattern to remain in utero without its suffering any permanent damage. The clinician now has very little by way of objective information to help assess what is happening to the fetus, particularly in a dynamically changing phenomenon such as labor. Timing intervention is all too often intuitive.

Dr. Friedman: One has to put fetal surveillance into the context of labor progression as well. Whereas the fetus may not be hypoxic at any given moment (as demonstrated by a normal heart rate pattern), we cannot rest confident that vaginal delivery will occur or even that it should occur. The issue of fetal wellbeing cannot be separated completely from that of obstetric management, of course, but we must not be deluded into complacency about the feasibility of a fetus delivering through the pelvis without damage merely because the heart rate monitoring record shows a normal pattern for the moment. Take for example the patient in whom you have uncovered an arrest disorder of labor progress (by dilatation and descent graphs). Here it becomes mandatory to rule out cephalopelvic disproportion before allowing the labor to proceed further because the combination of such a major labor dysfunction with disproportion generally demands that cesarean section be done. Regardless of the fetal condition, documentation of disproportion provides justification for proceeding immediately with cesarean section. In the absence of disproportion, further labor can be permitted—usually with uterotonic stimulation—provided the fetus will tolerate it. Here the further trial of augmented labor will usually be acceptable as long as there is clear evidence that there is no adverse effect on the fetus, particularly as regards the development of late deceleration patterns on the monitor. The point is that both factors—labor progression patterns in conjunction with cephalopelvimetric assurances and fetal heart rate patterns—must be considered separately.

Dr. Seitchik: We have to avoid tunnel vision when assessing a labor problem. If the fetus is doing well, we cannot ignore the developing abnormal labor. If labor appears to be obstructed, merely because the fetus is continuing to do well on the monitor does not justify subjecting it to possible mechanical damage from oxytocin stimulation.

Dr. Noah: The issue of a means for adequately adjudging cephalopelvic relations has been raised. Are there reliable techniques? Is this a subject for profitable future research endeavors?

Dr. Friedman: Our current approach consists of a series of evaluations beginning with clinical examination of the patient's pelvic architecture and dimensions early in pregnancy and again before and during labor, progressing to close observation of the dilatation and descent patterns as indices of suspicion to identify the women who are most likely to manifest disproportion, followed in designated cases with a dynamic assessment of fetal thrust as well as x-ray cephalopelvimetry. The dynamic test (so-called Müller-Hillis maneuver) involves a vaginal examination late in the course of labor, at the height of a contraction with added fundal pressure applied, in order to determine whether the fetal head is tightly fixed in the pelvis or will descend further. The thrust thus observed is a good measure of fit. As to x-ray techniques, I firmly hold that if the procedure is unable to provide accurate measurement of the fetal head regardless of its position or presentation, it should not be done. I feel it is unacceptable to radiate the fetus merely to obtain pelvic measurements which by themselves give very little clinically useful information about the adequacy of that pelvis to accommodate that particular fetus in that patient at that time in her labor. We utilize the Ball technique exclusively because it is simple, reproducible, and accurate, and will expose the fetus and maternal gonads to minimal radiation (only standing anteroposterior and lateral films taken at a measured distance are required). Certain critical measurements of pelvic diameters and fetal head circumference are obtained and corrected for distortion by simple triangulation methods. This provides an objective and reliable means for determining the relationship between fetus and pelvis.

Unfortunately, there are no recent prospective studies to show the benefit of pelvimetry. Several retrospective reports have denigrated the practice—with justification, criticizing those techniques which fail to measure the head as being inadequate to provide clinically useful information to help in meaningful decision-making. There is overriding need to subject the more relevant Ball technique to objective evaluation. Those using it usually act on their findings, of course. Therefore, it becomes impossible to use retrospective data to evaluate the efficacy of the method as a predictor of the outcome because the method has perforce influenced the results. Whether controlled prospective studies can be done ethically is unresolved.

Dr. Kriewall: The development of medical technology in this area is crisis-oriented. It has as its prime objective the diagnosis of abnormality. Physiology is obviously important and seems to be overlooked in general. Perhaps we should direct our attention toward development of medical instrumentation to study various physiologic parameters that may show us how the cervix or the uterus works or how the fetus behaves under various conditions of labor or under various pharmacologic influences. Can we be imaginative, for example, in seeking measurable aspects of the labor process that would serve as prognostic indicators?

Dr. Friedman: This addresses the crux of our interest. Much of what has been discussed thus far has dealt, directly or indirectly, with this very issue. While we seek to quantitate uterine pressure, we realize it would be naive to consider it to be an exclusive end-point for the labor process. We need more sensitive and objective techniques for measuring such factors as cervical dilatation, effacement, and resistance, fetal station, fetopelvic relationships, and cranial molding as well. All can be integrated into a complex mechanism for study of the physiology of the normal labor phenomenon, determining not only the impact of various influences of uterine contractility and the expulsive forces, but the impact in turn of these forces on cervical changes, fetal descent, and deformation of the fetal cranial contents.

Additionally, we need a means for better on-line assessment of the fetal respiratory physiology as related to transplacental exchange mechanisms and how such mechanisms are affected by the labor process. There are some coarse aspects of fetal physiology that are almost within our grasp to monitor, including fetal breathing, movement, cardiac and urinary function, nutrition and growth, oxygenation, and acid-base status. Also, we are capable of measuring preciously few of the many functions that the placenta is recognized to have in its role of maintaining pregnancy, preparing the maternal reproductive system, and sustaining the fetus.

Without filling in the huge gaps in our current knowledge of the physiology of the complexities of the labor phenomenon, we will have to be content to continue our present crisis-oriented approach by which we merely make empirical diagnoses of impending catastrophe. Many of the diagnostic criteria upon which our present diagnoses are based appear to have been evolved almost exclusively from isolated clinical disasters that yielded depressed or damaged infants. This is hardly an adequate basis for knowledgeable therapeusis. Our needs are patently clear; the directions which future research activities should take to satisfy those needs remain to be more fully elucidated. We are optimistic that the work we have reviewed here may serve to guide us and others along productive pathways.

REFERENCE

1. Schifrin, B.D., and Dame, L. Fetal heart rate patterns: Prediction of Apgar score. *JAMA* 219:1322, 1972.

INDEX